Praise for
Living with Crohn's & Colitis

"This book is an essential resource for anyone diagnosed with Crohn's or colitis. The authors do an excellent job of explaining what we currently understand about the complex interactions between the gut, our immune and nervous systems, and the microbial environment. The whole body approach to achieving wellness and the personal experiences of Dede Cummings make this book uniquely positive and offer the newly diagnosed patient the tools to help themselves on the path to balance and health."

—Kimberly Allison, M.D., author of the forthcoming book, *Red Sunshine*, and director of Breast Pathology at the University of Washington in Seattle

"Dede is an amazing woman! In this book you will find not only helpful advice but real inspiration."

—Julie Silver, M.D., assistant professor, Harvard Medical School, author of *What Helped Get Me Through: Cancer Survivors Share Wisdom and Hope*

"*Living with Crohn's and Colitis* is wonderfully written and rich with natural healing solutions for these all-too-common illnesses."

—Peter D'Adamo, N.D., author of *Eat Right for Your Type*

"I believe Dede's success rests on the fact that she incorporated such a comprehensive approach to managing her health. Dede remained fully committed to her plan throughout the ups and downs of her disease. She never gave up. Her positive attitude and tenacity helped her stick to the plan even when it was difficult. When an individual carries a chronic disease diagnosis, they must make themselves and their health the highest priority. Her journey with Crohn's will hopefully inspire others to make the difficult but rewarding choices to achieve health."

> —Renee Lang, N.D., Cancer Treatment Centers
> of America, Eastern Regional Medical Center,
> Philadelphia, Pennsylvania

"As a naturopathic physician, I recognize the myriad reasons patients seek integrative care. Patients who chose complementary medicine as a first line approach to their health issues have decided to follow a direction they believe is appropriate for their situation . . . despite outside influences . . . which pressure them to remain only in the mainstream.

Many individuals come to "alternative" medicine because conventional medical treatments are no longer working. They often arrive at the practitioner's office in a depleted, exhausted and desperate state after many failed medical regimens and procedures. They may appear disempowered and hopeless, a state of mind extremely detrimental to their health. In addition, there is the patient group who feels that they can chose from the best of both worlds—traditional treatments if necessary and the wide range of proven and effective non-conventional models of care that are accessible. It would be ideal if this choice were available at the beginning of their healthcare journey. . . . This book is a great resource."

> —Samantha K. Eagle, N.D., Medical Director,
> Biologic Integrative Healthcare,
> Brattleboro, Vermont

LIVING WITH
CROHN'S &
COLITIS

LIVING WITH
CROHN'S &
COLITIS

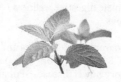

A Comprehensive Naturopathic Guide
for Complete Digestive Wellness

Jessica Black, N.D.
& Dede Cummings

》 hatherleigh

Hatherleigh Press is committed to preserving and protecting the natural resources of the Earth. Environmentally responsible and sustainable practices are embraced within the company's mission statement.

Hatherleigh Press is a member of the Publishers Earth Alliance, committed to preserving and protecting the natural resources of the planet while developing a sustainable business model for the book publishing industry.

Library of Congress Cataloging-in-Publication Data
    Black, Jessica.
    Living with Crohn's & colitis : a comprehensive naturopathic
    guide for complete digestive wellness / Jessica Black and
    Dede Cummings.
       p. cm.
    Includes bibliographical references and index.
    ISBN 978-1-57826-341-7 (pbk. : alk. paper)
    1. Inflammatory bowel diseases--Popular works. I.
    Cummings, Dede. II. Title.
    RC862.I53B53 2010
    616.3'44--dc22
                 2010017863

All Hatherleigh Press titles are available for bulk purchase, special promotions, and premiums. For information on reselling and special purchase opportunities, call 1-800-733-3000 and ask for the Special Sales Manager.

Interior design by Carolyn Kasper, DC Designs
Cover design by Nick Macagnone

))) hatherleigh

www.hatherleighpress.com

20 19 18 17 16 15
Printed in the United States

blessing the boats
(at St. Mary's)

may the tide
that is entering even now
the lip of our understanding
carry you out
beyond the face of fear
may you kiss
the wind then turn from it
certain that it will
love your back   may you
open your eyes to water
water waving forever
and may you in your innocence
sail through this to that

—Lucille Clifton (1936–2010)

DEDICATION

Dede

To my family and friends, especially Sam, Emma, and Joey; and to Steve for being there for me when I needed him.

Jessie

To my family, staff, and patients for being so understanding of my deadlines and for continuing to help me grow passionately as a physician, mother, and wife.

CONTENTS

PART II: Living with IBD

PART III: Recipes for Wellness:
How to Reduce Inflammation Through Diet

PREFACE

THE GREAT majority of books about inflammatory bowel diseases are written by physicians and scientists, and most are focused on a purely allopathic disease model. *Living with Crohn's and Colitis* sets itself apart from the rest with its thorough discussion of the many dimensions to this complex disease. The book offers a treatment regimen that encompasses the mind, lifestyle, and food intake, offering a concept of wellness and a plan for better living, not just temporary remission of the inflammatory process.

Today, massive research efforts are underway to unravel the biological underpinnings of the "universe" of some 100 trillion microorganisms that inhabit our gut, in order to better understand the role they play in triggering chronic gut inflammation. Many factors are major players in the development and persistence of such debilitating diseases like ulcerative colitis and Crohn's disease. New therapies offer help for all patients with these conditions, including those who were previously resistant to conventional therapies with anti-inflammatory drugs; these patients often ended up with multiple bowel resections and intractable fistulas. *Living with Crohn's and Colitis* studies the complexities of these interactions and takes other influences on these systems into consideration, presenting a comprehensive discussion of major factors in the development and persistence of ulcerative colitis and Crohn's disease.

Living with Crohn's and Colitis presents two different perspectives, the subjective experience of an insightful and well-informed patient, Dede, and the authoritative knowledge of complementary treatment approaches to conventional medical therapy, through Dr. Black. The authors present a holistic model of disease and wellness that takes into account not only the specific disease mechanisms and cutting-edge therapies, but also the interconnectedness of mind and body, of different organs with each other, and of a lifestyle in harmony with oneself and with one's environment. The ultimate goal is not remission but wellness. While Dr. Black provides an impressive overview of the current state of scientific knowledge about the pathophysiology and medical treatment options, as a naturopathic doctor, she also introduces concepts about alternative and complementary treatment options which rarely are offered to patients in the traditional medical setting. This makes *Living with Crohn's and Colitis* a unique source of information which should be an obligatory reading assignment for every patient suffering from inflammatory bowel disease.

In many ways, *Living with Crohn's and Colitis* is a book closely linked with recent medical study. Emerging scientific evidence clearly supports a holistic (or sometimes referred to as a "biopsychosocial") model of disease pathophysiology and therapy of all chronic diseases, including inflammatory bowel diseases. While the nervous system and its intricate connections with the gut-based immune system, and the likely interactions between the trillions of bacteria and the nervous system (the "brain gut microbial axis") are not mentioned in the great majority of text books and research articles on IBD, recent evidence clearly supports an important role of such neuroimmune interactions in disease activity and recurrence. Recent well-designed epidemiological studies have "rediscovered" the association of psychosocial stressors, depression and anxiety with relapse rates and disease severity. It remains unknown if this association reflects simply a role of the mind in modulating the disease processes, an influence of chronic gut inflammation on brain regions concerned with the modulation of mood and affect, or—most likely—a combination of both.

Still, there is much work to be done. Considering the fact that mediators of the central stress system (in particular the corticosteroids) have remained one of the most effective treatments for IBD, it is remarkable that not a single well-designed study has been undertaken to evaluate the possible role of alterations in the body's own steroid signaling as an important factor in disease modulation. The dramatic progress in unraveling the biological underpinnings of the nervous system, both the brain and enteric nervous system (often referred to as the "second brain"), has gone nearly unnoticed by experts and clinicians in the field of IBD, despite the fact that these breakthroughs have occurred in such areas as psychoneuroimmunology, affective neuroscience, stress neurobiology and in research areas looking at the biological effects of sleep and exercise on mood, affect, and well being. Additionally, nutrition and lifestyle have not been considered important elements of the disease process, even though concepts such as the "hygiene hypothesis" have reintroduced our surroundings and how we interact with these surroundings as possible central factors in the pathophysiology of IBD and other autoimmune disorders. Finally, the concept of *wellness*, e.g. not just "the absence of gut inflammation," has been a totally foreign concept to the majority of scientists. Change may not be far off, however, as the unraveling of the neurobiological underpinnings of positive mood states progresses. Currently, the idea that the subjective experience of wellness may reflect the conscious awareness of the myriad of body signals the brain receives every moment has moved the concept of wellness from the "touchy feely" realm of holistic gurus into the field of health psychology. *Living with Crohn's and Colitis* carefully considers the relationship between psychological processes and the immune system and many other factors influencing disease and wellness.

The coauthors of *Living with Crohn's and Colitis*, Dede Cummings and Dr. Black, have done a remarkable job of providing a comprehensive account of the patient's complex interactions with the medical system. *Living with Crohn's and Colitis* "fills in the holes" within the traditional medical framework of disease by providing a step-by-step approach to using specific complementary treatments in conjunction with traditional treatments. Traditional treatments range from specific recipes to herbal supplements to the evaluation of such mind-based approaches as yoga and mindfulness meditation. Through this approach, Dede and Dr. Black have created a framework for patients to become active players in the path to wellness, not just passive recipients of ever more sophisticated medical therapies. Despite our current scientific ignorance about specific effects of herbs and nutrients, as well as body postures and breathing techniques, this book allows the patient to partly take charge of their own management so he or she can feel empowered and confident of the outcome of their condition. While many of these holistic concepts have their origins in ancient healing traditions, including the Aryuvedic and traditional Chinese medicine traditions, *Living with Crohn's and Colitis* may in fact be a blueprint for a new medical approach to IBD management in the not too distant future.

EMERAN A. MAYER, M.D.
Director, UCLA Center
for Neurobiology of Stress
Division of Digestive Diseases
Los Angeles, California

FOREWORD

IT IS WITH pride and pleasure that I write this foreword for *Living with Crohn's and Colitis*, the new book from Dede Cummings and Dr. Jessica Black, which offers new and important insights about the best choices in integrative care, specifically naturopathic treatments for these chronic and often vexing forms of inflammatory bowel disease. The authors provide a wealth of insight into often underappreciated strategies that may allow those challenged by inflammatory bowel disease to take charge of their own destiny. Using these strategies may allow any reader to become what physicians call the "exceptional patient"—the individual who derives the maximum benefit by utilizing the combination of inspired medical advice and diligent self-care.

What I find particularly attractive about this book is how it integrates personal experience with medical knowledge. The first chapter profiles co-author Dede Cummings' experiences as a lifelong Crohn's disease patient. Dede, an award-winning book designer, writes engagingly and poignantly about her struggles with Crohn's and her voyage of self-discovery and healing that culminates in her hiking the "Long Trail" (the length of Vermont) in one-week sections, finally realizing a long-term goal that had been put off due to illness.

The book is also a terrific nuts-and-bolts guide of basic nature cure for inflammatory bowel disease. Jessica Black is one of those bright new lights in naturopathic medicine who can translate her passion for science into a passion for people. We might well consider her a *fundamentalist* of sorts. Her advice is grounded in the basics of naturopathic technique and philosophy: A cleansing balancing of the body's internal environment and the promotion of proper organ function. The goal here is to reverse the disease process, not just try to treat symptoms.

However, make no mistake. Dr. Black knows her science. The sections on inflammation, immunity, and the gut are as complete and thorough as anything I have yet encountered. What marks it as special is Jessica's dexterity in distilling the complexities of the immune system and its role in inflammatory bowel disease into a highly readable primer for the average person.

Perhaps most extraordinary, for a science-based book of this sort, is just how much emphasis is given to the connection between mind and body. Dr. Black sees much of the treatment of inflammatory bowel disease as boundary issues of a sort requiring both a physical and emotional approach. As she writes, "I think of the gut as our initial boundary protecting us from the outside world. A compromised gut is often connected with compromised emotional boundaries." Those of us who have been in practice long enough to have seen a requisite number of inflammatory bowel disease patients know well the truthfulness of this approach.

Living with Crohn's and Colitis is highly prescriptive. However, those looking for hope in a shoebox of supplements will probably come away disappointed. Those readers worried that by embarking on a naturopathic approach they might compromise their conventional medical care can rest assured. This is an integrated, broadly based approach. In fact, it is the concerted actions of all schools of healing that most often yield the best results, and *Living with Crohn's and Colitis* is the reader's best guide to this successful approach.

The book concludes with a simple three-month plan that is designed to transport the reader from disease to health. The suggestions are well paced and practicable. I especially appreciated the inclusion of a maintenance plan because in health, just like in sailing, "it is easier to stay dry than it is to get dry." Helpful recipes and carefully selected resources round out the book.

The word *doctor* is derived from the original Latin *docere*, which means "to teach." Sadly we do very little teaching in our modern day disease care system, preferring to park the ambulance at the foot of the cliff rather than at the precipice. Yet this book provides you with the opportunity to do something that no health care facility can do for you: Convert private time into therapy time. Expand that outwards over the years, months and days, and you have a road map to an exceptional outcome.

I once knew a famous choreographer who told me, "Forty percent of any dance is the ending." Modern science is still trying to decipher the mystifying reasons why a person might develop inflammatory bowel disease. Genes, infections, and hypersensitivity probably all play their part, and prevention on these levels may still lie in the future. However, I believe the book that you now hold in your hands contains the wisdom sufficient for you to end your dance on a high note.

PETER D'ADAMO, N.D.
Author, *Eat Right For Your Type*
Wilton, Connecticut

NOTE TO
THE READER

YOU MAY be wondering, of all the books available today on digestive disorders, what sets this one apart?

The answer is simple: *you.*

Whether you are living with it yourself or are a relative, caregiver, or loved one of someone with the condition, *Living with Crohn's and Colitis* is meant to be a comprehensive guide and a tool for wellness that can be personalized for your specific needs. In fact, *Living with Crohn's and Colitis* came into being when Dede, who was newly diagnosed with Crohn's disease, was searching for a book that would not only provide her with the information she needed about her condition, but also help her manage an incurable illness in a way that was best for her. When Dede couldn't find the book she needed, she and Dr. Black collaborated to write *Living with Crohn's and Colitis.*

This book is both a comprehensive guide to Crohn's and colitis, conditions that are part of a category known as inflammatory bowel disease (IBD), and a plan for wellness. Written thoughtfully with both the compassion and sensitivity offered by a lifelong Crohn's disease sufferer and a naturopathic physician, *Living with Crohn's and Colitis* provides a unique, patient-focused perspective and draws on both Western and alternative therapies to offer IBD sufferers help and hope for living fully.

In writing this book, it is our hope that you will be able to incorporate the information, tips, and plans for wellness into your own life. Ultimately, this book is yours to use as you feel is best.

A NEW LEASE ON LIFE

The journey that led to the creation of this book began with Dede's experience upon leaving the hospital in the spring of 2006. At that time, she had lived with a moderate case of Crohn's for eight years and had been in and out of the hospital four times for treatment of her flare-ups. She was ready to learn how to manage her condition and take a proactive role in her own health so that she could avoid more hospital stays, enjoy life, and do the things she loved again.

After returning home, Dede began to search for a book that would aid in her recovery and help her establish a "new lease on life." Surprisingly, she couldn't find this book anywhere—so she began writing a proposal to create the book she was looking for: a book that would be predominantly a wellness guide to living with an incurable disease.

In the office of her local naturopath, Dr. Renee Lang, Dede saw a book by another naturopath, Dr. Jessica Black. The book, entitled *The Anti-inflammation Diet and Recipe Book*, made its way into Dede's kitchen almost immediately, and she soon discovered that Dr. Black's delicious recipes were helping in her recovery and continued remission from Crohn's disease. Soon, Dede reached out to Dr. Black to thank her and propose that they collaborate on *Living with Crohn's and Colitis*: a patient-practitioner story that would serve as a guide for those with inflammatory bowel disease.

HOW THIS BOOK CAN HELP YOU

The intention of this book is to provide you with the most comprehensive and well-researched treatment options for inflammatory bowel disease (the suggestions in this book can also be applied to various gastrointestinal illnesses) so that you can use this knowledge to develop a treatment plan that works for you. *Living with Crohn's and Colitis* provides sound scientific explanations of why disease occurs and how to prevent or reverse the disease process. In

addition to providing the facts and most common treatment suggestions, this book looks at some alternative therapies that have proven
effective for many. You will find ample suggestions for lifestyle and
diet changes in addition to a comprehensive section guiding you
through the emotional ups and downs often experienced with these
diseases. No matter how busy you are, *Living with Crohn's and Colitis*
will fit into your life. The collection of information and advice for
various conditions has been designed to be easily applied to living a
full and healthy life in today's fast-paced world.

ABOUT US

What sets this book apart is that we empathize with you. We know
what it is like to suffer from illness, and we want to help you regain
wellness.

Dede's perspective—the patient's perspective—makes this book
unique and personal. Through her story, you will learn how she
became an advocate for herself upon receiving her Crohn's diagnosis. As the years have gone by and Dede has developed a better understanding of her body and its healing, she has become a
resource for alternative therapies. To date, she has been a co-speaker
with gastroenterologist Jeffry Potash, M.D., and surgeon Thomas
H. Lewis, M.D., at Brattleboro Memorial Hospital, and Corey A.
Siegel, M.D., director of the Inflammatory Bowel Disease Center at
Dartmouth-Hitchcock Medical Center, where Dede helps to further
the mission of helping people balance their clinic treatments with
outside alternative therapies. For the past three and a half years,
Dede has remained in full remission by balancing a traditional
medical plan with a naturopathic treatment plan.

As a naturopathic doctor, Dr. Jessica Black draws upon her years
of training and practice to present a well-rounded study of inflammatory bowel disease and how to manage and resist disease in order
to achieve a balanced, healthy lifestyle. Naturopathic doctors use a
holistic and preventative approach to healing that combines safe and

effective traditional therapies with the most up-to-date advances in modern medicine. Naturopathic medicine is an appropriate and effective treatment for a broad range of health conditions affecting people of all ages because methods and modalities are selected and applied based upon the individual needs of the patient.

In combining the voice of a patient and the perspective of a doctor, we hope to offer you a better understanding of how to live with Crohn's and ulcerative colitis whether you have one of these diseases or are a relative or caregiver of an IBD patient.

OUR HOPE FOR YOU

Our motive is primarily to help others who suffer—silently, in many cases—from an inflammatory bowel disease. If, by reading our book, a patient feels supported, educated, and empowered (all good things that aid in recovery) then we will have succeeded in our mission to write a book that will be groundbreaking in the area of wellness and recovery for those patients.

It is our hope that with this resource you can change your health and your future. Remember, the number one change you can make is your mindset. Believe in change, believe in yourself and your body's ability to heal, and believe you can be well and live well.

PART I

Understanding
Inflammatory Bowel Disease

CHAPTER 1
Dede's Story

I WAS 45 when I learned about the disease that was going to change my life. Up until then, my life had been largely without significant personal struggle. As an adult, I had celebrated the birth of three healthy babies and enjoyed a career that I loved, working in the world of book publishing. Some travel, fluency in another language, a college degree, and an outwardly happy family formed the nucleus around a marriage to my college boyfriend. Under the surface were family tensions and the death of one of my closest friends, a doctor, from breast cancer at the age of 41, which left me confused and somewhat prone to depression. As will be evident in this story, however, I masked the pain of emotional distress and physical trauma quite well. Ultimately, although this book is mainly about disease and recovery, it is also about confronting pain courageously and living life to celebrate it.

The year of my diagnosis was a busy one for me and my family. My husband Steve was taking a yearlong leave of absence from his college teaching job to design and build our house with a small crew. I was financially responsible for our young family during that time, and I was focused on starting my business—a small graphic design and consulting firm that specializes in book publishing design and packaging.

Buying land and building our house had long been a dream of ours. Steve and I had planned this phase for a year beforehand.

Now we were finally doing it! The year was obviously a stressful one for us all, but it was also very exciting. By December 2000, we were moved in and things began to return to normal. But in the spring of 2001, I injured both my knees playing on a women's softball team and had knee surgery in July. By early September, I was still on crutches. My knees were not healing as fast as they should have—I was demoted to the "pool" in physical therapy, a place filled with old people walking back and forth in the shallow end as fast-paced swimmers used the laps as if taunting us "PT-people." Despite this setback, I continued my usual daily routines. After bringing the children to school, I worked an eight-hour day, came home and fixed dinner, did laundry, washed the dishes—and then finally collapsed on the couch after another typical day! I allowed myself little opportunity for socializing or relaxation practices such as yoga or mediation—there simply wasn't time. I often skipped lunch and avoided exercise due to my bad knees and healing problems. Mostly, I was run down and not drinking enough water or getting enough sleep to deal with being run down. Certainly, my high carbohydrate diet was not helping at all.

During this time, I began teaching a college course in graphic design and was busy getting our kids ready for a new school year. We were still finishing our new house and stress levels were high. Over the long Labor Day weekend, I began to throw up frequently, and by September 9th of 2001, I was quite sick and unable to keep any food or water down. I called my doctor that night, and she said to get to the emergency room as quickly as possible.

I remember vividly that my husband had to carry me out the door and, as we left the house, our then twelve-year-old daughter Emma asked if this was going to be fatal. I had never realized that the kids were actually paying that much attention to me and what was happening. I felt heartbroken that we had to leave them in the care of our neighbor for the evening.

I was admitted to our small-town hospital. It was a Sunday evening, and the place was crowded. I was put in a bed, and I remember noticing that my roommate had a perforated bowel due to a colonoscopy that had gone wrong—not a good sign! I was feeling tired, scared, and alone—feelings that, although I did not know it then, were common for sufferers of Crohn's disease and ulcerative colitis. I would soon learn that, among other things, my potassium and other vital nutrients were depleted—typical problems from which IBD patients suffer.

A nurse came in and started an IV I was in a tremendous amount of pain, and I was scared, which only added to the cycle of pain and tension. The nurse was probably bummed out that it was late in the evening and that she had to administer an IV just as her shift was ending. She had a hard time with it due to my dehydration. When the tube was in, I immediately complained of "burning" and "pain." She rolled her eyes, looked at my husband conspiratorially, and said, "She's just tired, don't worry!" And with that, she left, and my husband went home to be with our children. I lay in the bed, moaning. The pain progressed up my arm, and I buzzed the nurse. My nurse came back in, she huffed and puffed, and then administered a bit of lidocaine to help with the pain. I cried and begged her to get her supervisor. When the supervisor came, she immediately took out the tube, easing the pain of infiltration. After the supervisor administered an IV in my other arm, I slept like a baby.

During my stay at the hospital, they gave me fluids and potassium to balance the electrolytes lost due to vomiting. The surgeon put me on a program called "bowel rest," during which time the patient receives nothing by mouth other than ice chips until things settle down. It worked quite well and they said I could go home on Tuesday morning.

I remember being taken down to have an X-ray done early on Tuesday morning. The X-ray was to determine if the pockets of air in my small bowel had continued to abate, which would further justify releasing me along with the joyous occasion of flatulence which would further bolster my case. I did not want to have surgery. Most of all, I wanted the oatmeal that the nurses had promised me after my X-ray.

After the X-ray, I was returned to my room. My surgeon sat upon my bed wearing his white hospital robe and looking strangely undignified. I thought how odd it was to see this surgeon sitting atop my covers, and I felt embarrassed that my bed wasn't properly made. As I drew closer, I noticed that he was staring up at the TV screen with what looked like a tear coming down the side of his cheek.

He was watching the Twin Towers being attacked on live television. It was 9/11.

Because it was within 10 miles of a nuclear power plant, the entire hospital was in evacuation/hazmat/emergency mode. No one even looked into my room to check on me that morning. Not knowing how to change the controls on my television, I sat in my bed watching the airplanes hit the towers over and over.

Later that week, a CAT scan revealed that I did indeed have Crohn's disease. From that day on, my life changed forever.

This book is my story, but it is also a way for Dr. Black and I to aid others who are either newly diagnosed with this lonely and debilitating disease or who have a loved one who is living with the disease. It is our hope that no matter what challenge you face today, reading this book will provide you with hope and lead you to a brighter future.

CHAPTER 2

An Introduction to Crohn's Disease and Ulcerative Colitis

ACCORDING TO Steven Bensen, M.D., Dede's gastroenterologist at Dartmouth-Hitchcock Medical Center in Hanover, New Hampshire, *Crohn's disease* and *ulcerative colitis* (often called colitis or UC for short) are on the rise across the board in the United States. These diseases are common among both men and women and have a strong genetic inheritance: nearly 20% of individuals diagnosed with Crohn's or colitis have a family member with the disease. There are approximately 1.5 million people with IBD in the United States alone, including 140,000 children, and that number has been steadily growing.

What are Crohn's disease and ulcerative colitis? These diseases are part of a category of illnesses known as *inflammatory bowel diseases* (IBD). *Inflammatory bowel disease (IBD)* is the general name for diseases that cause swelling in the intestines. IBD stems from a confusion in the immune system of the body's intestine. When this confusion occurs, the intestinal lining attacks normally harmless bacteria and inflammation follows (hence the name "inflammatory bowel disease").

According to the National Digestive Diseases Information Clearinghouse, "Crohn's disease is an inflammatory bowel disease. Because the symptoms of Crohn's disease are similar to other

WHAT'S THE DIFFERENCE BETWEEN INFLAMMATORY BOWEL DISEASE AND IRRITABLE BOWEL SYNDROME?

Crohn's and ulcerative colitis, which are the most common forms of inflammatory bowel disease, are not the same thing as *irritable bowel syndrome (IBS)*. IBS is a disorder of the lower intestinal tract that can cause cramping, diarrhea, bloating and pain. The cause of IBS is also unknown but, compared to IBD, IBS symptoms are more closely linked to the brain and emotional stress resulting in alternating diarrhea and constipation largely driven by emotional factors.

intestinal disorders, such as irritable bowel syndrome and ulcerative colitis, it can be difficult to diagnose." Crohn's disease (named for a Dr. Crohn who was part of a study circa 1932) is an inflammation of the transmural wall of the intestines, usually of the small intestine, but inflammation may involve any part of the GI tract.

Ulcerative colitis (UC) is characterized by mucosal ulceration in the colon where it causes inflammation and ulcers in the top layer of the lining of the large intestine. In contrast, for those with Crohn's disease, all layers of the intestine may be involved, and normal healthy bowel can be found between sections of diseased bowel.

THE ROLE OF THE IMMUNE SYSTEM

All inflammatory bowel diseases, including Crohn's disease and ulcerative colitis, are *immunologic-response* or *autoimmune diseases*. An *immunologic-response* or *autoimmune disease* is defined by an abnormal response of the immune system. In the case of Crohn's and UC, an immune response or defense mechanism is triggered as a result of something such as an environmentally-related cause. Suddenly, the immune system becomes overactive and damage to the body results. For individuals with Crohn's and UC, a variety of health issues can result.

A compromised immune system, resulting in inflammatory bowel disease, can lead to ancillary disorders of the eyes, liver, gallbladder, muscles and joints, kidneys and skin. In some cases, a fistula (an abnormal connection between two organs, characteristic of Crohn's disease but not ulcerative colitis) can form aberrant passages from your bowels to your anus, vagina, or skin surface.

WHAT CAUSES CROHN'S AND UC?

People with Crohn's and UC have abnormalities in their immune systems. What causes this? Currently, it is not clear, and there is no cure for these conditions.

Heredity has been thought to play a role in malfunctions of the immune system, perhaps triggered by something in the environment, brain, or an invading pathogen to the gut. Additionally, other theories based on recent research have proposed specific causes for Crohn's and UC, but no definitive answer has yet been discovered.

We will take a closer look at possible causes for Crohn's and UC, as well as the differences between the conditions, in Chapter 3. We will also discuss how the immune system plays a role in the onset of IBD in further detail.

Dede's Experience

Though I have never been clear about what caused my disease, there is a fair amount of ulcerative colitis and diverticular disease in my family history in addition to colon cancer.

I remember being told I had irritable bowel syndrome by my family doctor when my children were very small. At the time, I told him that a few people in my family had this condition and I didn't have time to worry about it. I now wonder whether I could have avoided a long and painful slide into disease had I embarked on Dr. Black's program for health and wellness or made an appointment with a gastroenterologist earlier.

As for environmental factors, I do remember being afflicted with food poisoning while vacationing on Cape Cod with my young family and friends in 1997. I began having more severe symptoms than irritable bowel syndrome after this time.

CAN CROHN'S AND UC BE PREVENTED?

Can proper nutrition and a healthy lifestyle lower the risk of developing Crohn's or UC? Some nutritionists think so. An improvement in lifestyle can help prevent "leaky gut," a condition that often leads to Crohn's, UC and other forms of IBD.

WHAT IS "LEAKY GUT"?

Known by doctors by its technical term, "intestinal permeability," this condition can encourage Crohn's disease, ulcerative colitis, irritable bowel syndrome (IBS), and other intestinal ailments in the IBD category. "Leaky gut" is a condition caused by inflammation of the gut lining. According to Andrew Weil, M.D.,

> "Leaky gut syndrome is not generally recognized by conventional physicians, but evidence is accumulating that it is a real condition that affects the lining of the intestines. The theory is that leaky gut syndrome (also called

increased intestinal permeability), is the result of damage to the intestinal lining, making it less able to protect the internal environment as well as to filter needed nutrients and other biological substances. As a consequence, some bacteria and their toxins, incompletely digested proteins and fats, and waste not normally absorbed may 'leak' out of the intestines into the blood stream. This triggers an autoimmune reaction, which can lead to gastrointestinal problems such as abdominal bloating, excessive gas and cramps, fatigue, food sensitivities, joint pain, skin rashes, and autoimmunity. The cause of this syndrome may be chronic inflammation, food sensitivity, damage from taking large amounts of nonsteroidal anti-inflammatory drugs (NSAIDS), cytotoxic drugs and radiation or certain antibiotics, excessive alcohol consumption, or compromised immunity."[1]

Leaky gut is more easily understood when learning that the lining of the gastrointestinal tract (the only tissue that separates the food contents of the stomach from the blood) is only about as thin as your eyelid. As inflammation increases due to damage, NSAID use, repetitive ingestion of food allergies, infection, and other insults, the tight junctions between cells of the gastrointestinal tract lining are affected and lose strength. As this happens, separation occurs between cells, resulting in larger tunnels in the GI lining. This, in turn, allows normally unauthorized and larger molecules to enter the blood stream. These chemicals are recognized as foreign by the immune system and immune complexes occur, resulting in confusion and autoimmune reactions against healthy tissue.

DIAGNOSIS

In many cases, inflammatory bowel diseases, including Crohn's and UC, are extremely difficult to diagnose. A plethora of symptoms abound, including cramping, diarrhea, bloating, nausea, vomiting, and bloody stool, making it difficult for both Western medical doctors and naturopathic doctors alike to diagnose.

In this book, *Western medicine* refers to medical doctors and nurses who treat disease symptoms through the use of drugs, surgery, and other medical interventions.

To arrive at a diagnosis, one of the first things a doctor does is take a complete medical history and order tests (for example, blood tests, colonoscopies, upper GI series tests such as barium enemas, and X-rays), if warranted. A genetic test may also be performed, and many naturopathic doctors will take stool samples. In addition, more and more traditional GI doctors are interested in exploring bacterial or parasitic causes for inflammation.

Given how complicated it is to diagnose IBD (especially Crohn's disease), patients are often left hanging for months or even years. Appendicitis is often confused with Crohn's because both conditions effect the location in the lower right quadrant of the abdomen. Ulcerative colitis is perhaps a bit easier to diagnose, as it is limited to the colon and is usually diagnosed with the aid of an instrument called an endoscopic camera during a routine *sigmoidoscopy* (where a tube is inserted into the rectum and travels through the large bowel while the patient is under sedation).

TREATMENT

The usual course of treatment is a step-by-step approach that corresponds to the waxing and waning aspects (also called "flare ups" in this book and in the medical world) of the patient's IBD, using medications such as aminosalicylate or cortiosteroidial drugs. If flare ups become more frequent, immunomodulatory drugs such as 6MP or azathioprine may be recommended. An alternative treatment is *Infliximab* (also known as Remicade). According to a recent lecture from Corey Seigel, M.D., director of the IBD clinic at Dartmouth-Hitchcock Hospital, these drugs will eventually become "designer drugs" that will be matched with a specific symptomatic form of IBD, with better patient outcomes.

Dede's Experience

After being diagnosed with Crohn's in 2001, I felt the need to have a second opinion, and I decided to go "right to the top" with Dr. Peter Banks, the director of the Clinical Gastroenterology Service at Brigham and Women's Hospital in Boston and an international authority in the field of pancreatitis. Dr. Banks has also been extremely active in conducting randomized prospective trials on newer treatments in inflammatory bowel disease.

Dr. Banks recommended I begin taking medication to slow the growth of scar tissue formation from my frequent flare-ups of Crohn's disease. He specified Purinethol 6MP, and/or another immunosuppressant drug, like Remicade, should be started immediately.

After my 2001 diagnosis, I went on a course of the antibiotic called Cipro for two weeks after my naturopath, Jody Noe, N.D., received the results of a stool sample she had ordered. Together with Dr. Jeffry Potash, my gastroenterologist, the naturopath worked with the doctor to proscribe a trial with the antibiotic, which worked remarkably well for a time.

SURGERY

In some cases of IBD, surgery might be necessary. Indications for surgery will be discussed later, but in most cases surgery occurs due to a life threatening problem, non-resolvable issue, or lack of response to oral therapy. Surgery to remove the large intestine is more common in patients with advanced ulcerative colitis. However, surgery for Crohn's disease is often not as straightforward. In many post-surgical patients, Crohn's disease recurs near the site of the first incision, making the odds for success less than desirable.

A good surgeon should be board-certified in colorectal surgery and a member of the Crohn's and Colitis Foundation of America. You should also look for a surgeon with a good (if not great) bedside manner because there are often major physical changes post-surgery (often as a result of adjusting to an internal pouch) and psychological adjustments to deal with, as well.

Dede's surgeon, Dr. Horace F. Henriques III, is a brilliant surgeon with capable hands and a sense of humor. He is a great example of a surgeon who goes to great lengths to make sure the pre-op and post-operative care is diligent and that the patient's outcome is favorable.

Dede's Experience

In the case of surgery, it is usually a last resort. In my case, I was extremely sick and really had no choice. There are different ways surgery can be performed, and patients should really consult with a surgical team, looking for a nearly unanimous decision before proceeding. Many UC patients end up having their colons removed by either having an ileostomy (a small opening is made after the colon is removed that attaches to a pouch, which can then be emptied) or other operations with variations of this technique.

In late May of 2006, I was scheduled for a bowel resection (a resection of the terminal ileum). I loved my surgical team, but I was very nervous and anxious the night before my operation. My naturopath created a pre- and post-surgical protocol using dietary supplements, homeopathic medicine, and medicinal herbs. For example, the herb arnica was used to help with post-operative pain management and is important in healing and recovery. Visual imaging also helped immensely. I meditated on the surgery with my own mantra:

White light healing river flow veins inflammation gone

I know this helped me. I just imagined the blood going away from the incision and the surgeon taking the disease out of me. I had a little bag of "talismans," including a photo of my three kids, holy water my Mom gave me from Lourdes, a small Buddha statue, an amulet from Tibet, and beads from Masaai women from Africa. They actually let me bring this bag in on my gurney, and it stayed right by my side the whole time. Also, I was quite impressed that my surgeon tried to find me an acupuncturist to help with my pain after the operation. This showed me how much my doctor was actually listening to me and seemed to go over and above the call of duty. I was lucky to have him, Dr. Horace Henriques, my hero.

When I got to the hospital, I brought my own bag with underwear, baggy pants to wear home, camisoles to wear under my hospital gown, my own slippers (a pair that is easy to slide in and out of), and even some hanging origami cranes and a framed photo of a botanical print by photographer Lynne Weinstein that I love to put on the wall.

Even though I used acupuncture to help with the pain after my surgery, I also used the Morphine pump, believe me! In recovery, I remember being so happy every time I could hear the resounding beep. My husband cracked up when I got this stupid grin on my face. You do have to wait something like 6 minutes between doses. Research suggests that these pumps allow patients to medicate themselves appropriately and the patient actually uses less pain medication by doing this.

A CD player or MP3 player with headphones is also a must for the hospital. I listened to classical music every morning (Brandenburg Concertos) and watched iPod videos like "Desperate Housewives"—all good distractions! Each night, I also listened to a meditation series called "Cultivating Compassion", which helped me to relax.

I also found talking to the nurses very informative and helpful. They will want you to "pass gas"—my nurses gave me "Smooth Move" Ayurvedic tea (by Traditional Medicinals), and that really helped me.

I walked around the hospital floors as much as I could, and with the help of a family member or friend, I was able to use a wheelchair to go outside for some fresh air and sun.

I went into the hospital on Monday, and my surgeon told me I could go home on Thursday. But I insisted on staying one more night. Stick up for yourself! If you don't feel ready to go home yet, let your doctors and nurses know.

After returning home from the hospital, I made sure to get lots of rest. I was careful not to pick up anything heavier than five pounds, and I avoided moving anything with my feet, as well. Ask friends or family to help out by cooking your family dinner every other night (you will have lots of leftovers) for the first two weeks. You can also reach out to church members, community members, co-workers, and other friends who you know and trust.

My husband and a friend set up a page for me on a site called "CaringBridge" (www.caringbridge.org), which is a free service that connects recovering patients with friends and family online. This proved to be a great outlet for me, my friends, and family. Even my office personnel got into it, and clients wrote to me!

MANAGING CROHN'S AND UC: THE POWER OF KNOWLEDGE

Although the causes of Crohn's, UC, and other forms of IBD are not clear, we do know that many of the associated symptoms can be relieved—and in some cases, eliminated—through various therapies and lifestyle modifications. For now there is no cure for Crohn's, UC, and IBD, but living a full life with these diseases is possible for anyone.

In the following chapters, we will take a closer look at what can exacerbate IBD, including food, chemicals, hormone, and lifestyle, and how having a greater understanding of these potential causes can help pave the path towards wellness.

Dede's Experience

What I have noticed in my later years—which, not co-incidentally, coincides with my quest for patient education and empowerment—is that many health care profession-als actually seek *me* out to ask me what I'm doing to stay so healthy. It seems that everyone knows someone who either has Crohn's or ulcerative colitis, and many are desperate for answers and guidance. For me, this was a real motivator in writing this book with Dr. Black; it seemed like the time was right to help people with IBD and other autoimmune diseases that are on the rise.

TOTAL HEALTH

For many people like Dede with Crohn's or UC, proactively guarding one's health and living can mean the difference between more time in the hospital and more time at home. In this book, you will find all the information you need to begin a thorough, effective plan for wellness that goes beyond drugs and surgeries.

There are many total-body health approaches that can ease the symptoms of IBD. Participating in a balanced treatment that includes the following might keep Crohn's disease at bay:

- acupuncture
- wheat-free, dairy-free and organic diet
- daily yoga and meditation
- massage and REIKI
- naturopathic treatment with probiotics
- GI management from traditional Western medicine with yearly colonoscopies and blood testing
- regular regimen of exercise
- psychotherapy
- physical therapy with integrative and cranial-sacral treatment

See Chapter 8 for more details on each of these treatments.

Dede's Experience

Working with a trusted doctor and/or naturopath helps to alleviate some of the fears of newly diagnosed IBD patients. Dr. Black and other naturopaths like Peter D'Adamo, N.D., are trail blazers in their approach to an allopathic model that combines many different modalities to help find a cure or at least help the patient lead a more full and productive life.

HOPE THROUGH RESEARCH AND SUPPORT

For anyone newly diagnosed with IBD, getting help with psychotherapy and talking in a support group are also vital to success.

Support groups can also be incredibly helpful. Organizations that support and fund research for both Crohn's disease and ulcerative colitis are strong and growing. The National Digestive Diseases Information Clearinghouse (NDDIC), along with the Crohn's & Colitis Foundation of America (www.ccfa.org) are both active in offering patients cutting edge research and studies, along with information on clinical trials.

Joining the membership of organizations related to your condition can be extremely helpful in obtaining valuable information and connecting with other individuals who have also been diagnosed.

DEFINING A NATUROPATHIC DOCTOR

A naturopathic doctor is one who practices a system of therapy that relies on natural remedies to treat illness by following a strict regimen of digestive enzymes, vitamins and other natural and herbal supplements.

Dede's Experience

I first joined the regional Crohn's & Colitis Foundation's chapter in Boston so that I could attend symposiums and find out about local clinical trials and developments. It was also a great resource for me to find my doctor. Because he was listed as a participating gastroenterologist, it gave me more confidence in choosing him. I call my membership in the CCFA my main "club," and it is with pride that I participate in some of their fundraising events to raise awareness and much-needed funds for research to find a cure for these insidious digestive diseases. As CCFA states on their website, "Whether you're newly diagnosed, have lived with Crohn's or colitis for years, or have a loved one who suffers from IBD, it's important to understand the impact of these diseases on day-to-day life."

YOUR ROAD TO WELLNESS

Again, the information presented in this book is not a definitive guide, nor does it present a cure. However, one major equation in overall success is patient participation, and you hold the key to your own best life. Having a positive attitude is key!

Dede's Experience

I remember when I was first diagnosed five years earlier, and I think back to the decision I made to follow a non-Western medical path. It is a path that has certainly been transformative, though not without pain or problems; it is a path that I would readily travel again.

In Robert Frost's seminal poem "The Road Not Taken," the poet speaks of burdens and traveling, as one who perhaps was long suffering, when he writes of the road less traveled: ". . . long I stood. And looked down one as far as I could . . ."

The "road to wellness" can take someone on a path that integrates naturopathic treatment with Western medicine. This is not a definitive guide or cure but a personal story which will hopefully help anyone who suffers from these insidious diseases.

As Dr. Black notes, "Everyone is different and may respond differently to the same exact therapies." This is eminently true. For example, I've met many patients through my support group at the hospital, through message boards and other social networking sites who say they cannot tolerate milk. On the contrary, I have no problem digesting lactose. Similarly, *Reiki*, a Japanese technique for stress reduction and relaxation that also promotes healing, did not work as well for me as did Integrative Manual Therapy, a treatment modality that assesses and treats pain and disease but uses the spinal cord to move the body's energy around. Perhaps Reiki was more diffuse and IMT, a more focused approach to pinpointing trauma within the body, worked better for me both physically and psychologically. There is more information about these treatments in Chapter 10: Lifestyle Guide for Reducing Inflammation and Promoting Digestive Health.

CHAPTER 3

Inflammatory Bowel Disease:
Immune Response, Inflammation,
and the Importance of Gut Health

THE INTIMATE encounter we have with the outside world begins in the stomach or the lungs. Every day we come in close contact with organisms from the outside world that can threaten our health. These foreign influences come into our bodies through the gastrointestinal tract and the mucus membranes of the lungs. In a healthy human, the internal mucus membranes in the gut and the lungs confront the invader as friend or foe, acting as the first line of defense against most invading micro–organisms. In the stomach or the lungs, the cells make up the *mucosal lining* that is integral and vital to the immune system.

THE IMMUNE SYSTEM AND THE GUT

The gut itself is an incredible system that covers a surface area nearly the size of a basketball court! Thus, a significant proportion of the body's immune system is found in the gastrointestinal tract. In the gastrointestinal lining, we have what is referred to as *GALT: gut associated lymphoid tissue*. GALT is essentially the gastrointestinal tract's immune system. As stated, the mucosal immune system in the gut works to protect us from foreign invaders that cause illness.

From a young age, the gastrointestinal tract is continually learning what types of foods it can tolerate and what types of foods and additives toward which it mounts "fighting" reactions. In this book, "oral tolerance" will be defined as the process of learning how not to react negatively to foods within the gastrointestinal tract. Building "oral tolerance" is different in each body and is dependent on many factors including genetics, one's physical and emotional environment, early food introduction, whether or not one was breast fed, proper balance of gastro-intestinal microflora, and the types of foods one ingests regularly. Oral tolerance will be discussed in more detail later in this chapter.

Imbalance within the immune system can alter the body's ability to maintain equilibrium of oral tolerance. In turn, the body starts mounting reactions against nutrient-rich foods, and no longer maintains a strong immunological reaction to foreign organisms that would normally cause disease.[1]

Whether you are aware of it or not, your gut plays a major role in overall immunity. In fact, autoimmune diseases, cancer, and all diseases associated with imbalanced immune response can relate in one way or another to the health of the gut. Simply said, the gastrointestinal tract and what we feed it, how we nurture it, and how it developed, cannot be ignored when approaching any illness holistically.

Terms like "gut tolerance," "bowel tolerance," or "oral tolerance" simply mean that the immune system has decided, as a team of specialized and sophisticated cells, to have no response to the foreign antigen. Oral tolerance is how we are able to eat many to most foods and not mount immunological reactions or impede the intake of needed nutrition.

> Scientists are not yet certain what causes Crohn's disease
> and ulcerative colitis, so they are known as *idiopathic dis-*
> *eases* or diseases with an unknown cause.

WHAT CAUSES INFLAMMATION?

As stated, *inflammatory bowel disease (IBD)* stems from a confusion, or misunderstanding, of the mucosal immune system function. When this confusion occurs, the intestinal lining can begin
mounting reactions against normally harmless bacteria, foods, etc.,
and inflammation occurs in the colon as a result.

The causes of inflammation for those with Crohn's, UC and
other forms of IBD are complex, involving a number of factors.
These include one's environment, microbial balance, genetics, stress
and emotional health, diet and lifestyle habits, and immunological
factors.

Although the cause of IBD, including Crohn's and UC, is not
clear, one can learn what causes inflammation for each individual,
and use this knowledge to improve lifestyle habits. We will take a
closer look at how managing these factors can help to control the
symptoms of Crohn's, UC and IBD in Part II.

MORE SYMPTOMS OF IBD

One of the main symptoms of IBD is inflammation, which can also
cause tissue damage, including ulceration, edema, bleeding, and
fluid and electrolyte loss.[2]

Other symptoms include:

- Frequent diarrhea, constipation, or both
- Abdominal cramps and severe pain
- Rectal bleeding
- Weight loss and fatigue
- Nausea and fever

DEDE'S MENTOR SPEAKS ABOUT LIVING WITH ULCERATIVE COLITIS

I was six months pregnant with my second daughter when I was diagnosed with ulcerative colitis. I had never heard of this disease before, but I sure learned a lot quickly! My first flare was fairly mild, and I thought that maybe this wouldn't be such a big deal. But a few months later, I found myself lying in a hospital bed for almost three weeks with an infant and a two year old at home, and I realized that my life had changed.

I came home, eventually got healthy, and focused on getting my life back. Educating myself about this disease was so helpful for me, and I was lucky enough to have an amazing support system. A big part of my support system was nutrition/hydration trainer Kate Devlin (whom I had gone to high school with) and she quickly introduced me to Team Challenge.

Less than two years after my diagnosis, I was at the Las Vegas Team Challenge starting line. What an amazing experience—the training, the relationships I formed, and then event weekend—my life had changed again, this time for the better. I am thrilled to be back this season as a mentor. I feel so lucky and proud to be a part of this team! I have loved meeting all of our new participants, and I hope that I can support all of them the way that I was so supported during my first season.

—BETHANNE PACKARD, *Dede's mentor and co-runner in the Boston Team Challenge ½ Marathon to benefit the Crohn's & Colitis Foundation*

A NOTE ON CELIAC DISEASE

According to the Celiac Disease Foundation (celiac.org), celiac disease is a lifelong, digestive disorder affecting children and adults. Like Crohn's and UC, celiac disease is not a food allergy; rather, it is an auto-immune disease. When people with CD eat foods that contain gluten, it creates an immune-mediated toxic reaction that causes damage to the small intestine and does not allow food to be properly absorbed. *Gluten,* from the Latin word for "glue," is the common name for proteins in specific grains. Even small amounts of gluten can affect those with CD and cause health problems. Damage can occur to the small bowel even when there are no symptoms present. Gluten that are harmful to persons with celiac disease are found in *all* forms of wheat (including durum, semolina, spelt, kamut, einkorn and faro) and related grains rye, barley and triticale and *must* be eliminated from their diet.

As in the case of the inflammatory bowel diseases in this book, celiac disease does not have a known cause. In 70% of identical twins, they both share the disease; this occurrence is the same for those with Crohn's (a stronger genetic risk than that of ulcerative colitis).

Note: Nearly all of the recipes in this book are gluten-free, and many of the suggestions in this book will be very helpful for this condition.

Dede's Experience

When people ask about my disease, I usually tell people I have "an immunologic (or autoimmune) disease triggered by environmental factors." That seems to work; they usually get the fact that I have a disease that is triggered by the immune system. When I define my disease to a stranger this way, we tend to avoid the awkward questions like, "Do you have diarrhea? Cramps? Vomiting?"

THE CHALLENGE OF DIAGNOSIS

The other difficulty that many readers, practitioners, and caregivers can appreciate is that Crohn's disease is hard to diagnose. In Dede's case, it masqueraded as conditions from ruptured ovarian cysts to appendicitis (Dede actually had ovarian laparoscopic surgery! Luckily, nothing was removed at that time).

The number one aspect of diagnosis is a proper and complete history. Many misdiagnoses would be spared if comprehensive histories could be taken by every physician. That being said, even with a comprehensive history and physical exam, the diagnosis can be overlooked, especially if common testing procedures are not utilized. Most physicians will use a combination of blood tests, endoscopies, X-rays, CAT scans or ultrasounds, and biopsies to help get a clear picture of the disease. By using these tests, many conditions can be ruled out as the cause of symptoms and results can reveal the diagnosis of inflammatory bowel disease.

TREATMENT

Historically, treatment options have been limited. Most conventional treatments focus on relieving symptoms with anti-inflammatory drugs or surgically removing the affected part of the intestines. Drugs that suppress the entire immune system are typically used to treat UC. Drug therapies that are typically used to treat severe cases include Aminosalicylates (Sulfasalazine and 5-ASA), corticosteroids (prednisone), immunomodulators (6MP), and other suppressive drugs similar to the drugs given to patients with Crohn's disease.

Our book is an attempt to suggest treatments for most people in a gentle, specific way that builds one treatment on top of another while understanding that everyone is different and may respond differently to each therapy. We offer many suggestions in this resource to suit the unique needs of each individual. As outlined in this book and as demonstrated through Dede's experience, there is promising new research that indicates greater hope for IBD sufferers who learn how to manage their lifestyle properly.

Dede's Experience

Post flare-ups and post-surgery, most people will likely experience good days and bad days. I remember being nervous about having to taper off of steroids after my bowel resection because I was worried that my disease would come back. When I got home from the hospital, I began tapering off of prednisone, which brought about a noticeable decline in my energy. To make up for this, I did my best to focus on all the friends and people who were supporting me. I also spent a lot of time reading and reflecting. A few books that helped me in my recovery was a series by Pema Chodron *Start Where You Are*, *The Places That Scare You*, and *When Things Fall Apart* published by Shambhala Publications.

INTERLEUKIN-23 AND IBD

New research has shown a genetic link to Crohn's disease and colitis through a gene called the interleukin-23 (IL-23) receptor. This supports what we already know about the significance of family history in IBD. Because interleukin-23 is a major cytokine in controlling gut inflammation, this information stresses the importance of reducing inflammation in the gut through controllable factors such as food choices, reducing stress, and promoting proper digestion.

AN OVERVIEW OF INFLAMMATION

In order to fully understand the symptoms and treatments for IBD, it is important to have a basic comprehension of how inflammation works within the body. Both inside and outside our bodies—including our intestines—inflammation plays an important role in maintaining health and wellness.

How does inflammation help to guard a healthy body? In a human being, inflammation is a response from the immune system that acts to protect and heal tissue within the body. For example, during times of invasion either by an insect bite, virus or bacteria, an injury, food allergy, or repetitive use of weight bearing joints, the immune system initiates inflammation as a signal in the body that cell repair and protection is needed.

In the case of a virus or bacteria invasion, immune cells directed at defeating the offending organism are sequestered to the area to act as the first line of defense in an effort to decrease the foreign invader's ability to spread throughout the body.

With a sprained ankle, the swelling, heat, and redness that you notice is a result of a direct and immediate inflammatory response whereby immune cells are sequestered to the area to help build and repair the area. The influx of immune cells and inflammation also serve to immobilize the joint so as not to cause further injury.

Finally, in the case of the gastrointestinal system, inflammation plays a role in regulating the impressive regulatory border. This allows the passage of some nutrients and chemicals and initiates a reaction to foreign chemicals that may pose harm.

A regulatory border within the body uses chemical messengers and hormones as keys to allow access to important chemicals and deny access to unwanted materials. The gastrointestinal tract is one of the most important regulatory borders we have in the body. It functions to allow healthful nutrients or beneficial bacteria in and to keep out unwanted microorganisms or larger food particles that may harm or overload the system.

The Process of Inflammation on a Cellular Level

There are a number of cells important in the inflammatory cascade.

The process of inflammation begins when the immune system triggers certain cells in the body, called leukocytes, to release *cytokines*. *Cytokines* may be *inflammation promoting* or *inflammation inhibiting*. Cytokines that promote inflammation stimulate the release of immune cells locally (to one area of the body) or systemically (throughout the whole body).

> Inflammation promoting cytokines include: TNF-alpha, interferon-gamma, interleukin-1, IL-6, and IL-12.[3] These will be discussed later in this chapter.

The cells that release cytokines are known as *Leukocytes*, or white blood cells; we generally think of them as our immune cells.

> ## SOME OF THE MAIN LEUKOCYTES INVOLVED IN INFLAMMATION ARE:
>
> - Monocytes that become macrophages (cells that engulf foreign invaders or material)
> - Mast cells
> - Neutrophils (cells that have enzymes inside allowing them to engulf a bacteria and neutralize it with the enzymes)
> - T-lymphocytes (cells that help to initiate and direct the immune response and form memory responses for future infections)
> - B-lymphocytes (cells that help to make antibodies needed for bacterial resistance)

> - NK cells (natural killer cells that kill viruses and bacteria by exocytosis of enzymes that have a direct effect on the invading organism)
> - Esosinophils (cells that function to defend against para-sites, though when the immune response is imbalanced and an elevation in esosinophils is present, allergies are often seen)

Leukocytes come in various forms, including lymphocytes and mast cells.

Leukocytes are the disease-fighters of the immune cells. They are produced and stored within the complex matrix of lymphatic tissue (see the box "The Lymphatic System" on page 33 for more details).

> Lymphocytes are the cells that are often out of balance in inflammatory diseases.

Another leukocyte of importance is the *mast cell*. The cytokines released by mast cells play the role of recruiting all of the other types of necessary white blood cells to the site where the body is being attacked. The result is an immediate and robust inflammatory response. In the case of an injured ankle, for example, the mast cells release the cytokines that cause the ankle to swell up in as little as a minute after injury occurs. Mast cells appear to be the primary white blood cell inflammatory mediator.

In addition to releasing cytokines, mast cells also secrete his-tamine. When a virus, bacteria, or a parasite invades the body, the cell begins a process known as exocytosis. Exocytosis occurs when the mast cells release into circulation inflammatory-promoting granules containing cytokines and histamine. *Histamine* plays an important role in initiating local immune responses. For example,

Histamine is responsible for the irritation and redness you notice around a swollen bug bite.

Histamines are also important to regulating physiological functioning within the gastrointestinal tract.

THE LYMPHATIC SYSTEM

The lymphatic system is comprised of the thymus gland, the spleen, the lymph nodes throughout the whole body, and the lymphatic tissue that lines the small intestine (called Peyer's patches, or aggregated lymphatic follicles which will be mentioned later). The lymphatic system gives birth to all of our important immune cells that were mentioned earlier. The T-lymphocytes thrive and mature in the thymus and the spleen hosts the red blood cells, some of the white blood cells, and plays a part in antibody manufacture. The lymphatic tissue and lymph nodes line every nerve and blood vessel in the body and function as our "highway" for immune cells and waste. Immune cells travel, repair, and fight, while wastes are eliminated constantly. The lymphatic system is continually moving wastes throughout the body and getting the wastes ready for export through main elimination organs such as the kidney, liver, gastrointestinal tract, and skin.

Making sure the lymphatic system is working properly is important in the treatment of all diseases—especially inflammatory bowel disease—because as we eliminate waste, it reduces stress on the elimination organs like the bowel, thereby supporting improved function. Accumulation of toxins in the bowel has a larger chance of confusing the immune response in inflammatory bowel disease patients.

Histamine stimulates blood vessels to allow larger quantities of white blood cells and proteins to pass through to an affected area and facilitate a successful attack on foreign invaders or stimulate the healing response during an injury.

This is why antihistamines can sometimes reduce inflammatory bowel disease symptoms; they reduce the body's allergic response and can eliminate the inflammation caused by food or other chemical reactions. This process will be discussed in more detail in the section on allopathic treatments (see page 105).

HISTAMINE AND ALLERGIES

Histamine is good at stimulating the body to react, but sometimes it is responsible for heightening the reaction to an exaggerated or pathological point. When histamine plays a part in hyper-reaction, it is referred to as an allergic reaction. Allergic reactions can vary in severity from mild to lethal.

INFLAMMATION AND IBD

In a healthy human being, inflammation serves an important, useful purpose in protecting the body from foreign invaders. But, as stated earlier, inflammatory bowel disease (IBD) stems from a confusion of the mucosal immune system function that results in extreme inflammation. Inflammation is a result of the intestinal lining mounting reactions against normally harmless bacteria, foods, etc.

According to the *American Journal of Gastroenterology*,[4] we learn that there is a direct relationship between the mucosal layer of cells and its interaction with contents in the intestine. In IBD, a misunderstanding in this relationship occurs that results in the intestine improperly stimulating pro-inflammatory cytokines and inhibiting anti-inflammatory cytokines. This results in active inflammation within the colon and, over time, tissue destruction if the pro-inflammatory cascade is left un-inhibited by balancing cytokines.

BACTERIAL INFECTION AND CROHN'S DISEASE: NEW THEORIES

Mycobacterium Para tuberculosis is being linked specifically to Crohn's disease. Mycobacterium Para tuberculosis is a type of mycobacterium usually associated with chronic *enteric* disease in domestic cattle, sheep, and goats (*enteritis* is a term referring to inflammation in the small intestine). It has long been suspected that a type of mycobacterium is a potential cause for Crohn's disease due to its association with chronic enteritis in animals. Research dating as far back as the 1990s has confirmed this suspicion and directly linked Mycobacteriaum Para tuberculosis with Crohn's disease manifestation. However, this bacterium does not seem to have a strong association with UC.

As mentioned earlier, minor insults may cause major upsets and shifts within the mucosal immune system resulting in the release of pro-inflammatory cytokines such as TNF-alpha (see Appendix A, page 261 for a detailed discussion on TNF), interferon-gamma (IFN-gamma), interleukin-1 (IL-1), IL-6,[5] and IL-12. In the continued presence of these inflammatory chemicals, tissue damage and destruction occurs. Without regulation of these pro-inflammatory cytokines, IBD is progressive and can worsen over time. The mucosal immune system of IBD sufferers is extremely sensitive and, in a sense, vulnerable due to a lack of down-regulating cytokines.

Because of this underlying mucosal immune problem, bacteria, virus, and parasites have an easy target in inflammatory bowel disease sufferers and this is why bacterial infections are often found in relation to IBD. Bacteria or viruses that cause infection within the gastrointestinal tract directly stimulate an inflammatory cascade. Often times in IBD sufferers, anti-microbial agents are used to treat symptoms if a bacterial etiology is suspected. A study published in the *American Journal of Gastroenterology*[6] supports the bacterial hypothesis by finding that plasma endotoxins (toxins released by bacteria) are more prevalent in IBD sufferers and may contribute to the increased inflammatory response and impairment of natural immunity in the intestine in IBD patients. Building on what we discussed earlier, intestinal contents that provoke an inflammatory response are most likely endotoxins released by particular kinds of bacteria in the gut. These bacteria may be opportunistic bacteria, probiotic bacteria, or foreign and pathogenic bacteria.

Contents in the intestine that cause reactions can be, but are not limited to, endotoxins from bacteria, food particles from regular foods that are not properly digested due to improper gastrointestinal tract functioning, or from food allergen particles.

Dede's Experience

In addition to a bout of food poisoning I had in 1997, I had also been treated in 1994 for an intestinal parasite called giardia, which I caught from swimming in the river near my home in southern Vermont. Early in 2001, my naturopath reviewed my stool sample lab results, which revealed an off-the-charts bacterial growth (and, unfortunately, not the beneficial kind of bacteria). I thought that my body had recovered from the food poisoning and the parasite, but the onset of Crohn's disease that culminated in the major flare-up of 2001 was perhaps linked to my infection, if in fact such a bacterial link existed.

Microrganisms exist in the body, as will be discussed later in the book. However, bad bacteria—like yeast, fungi, and parasites like giardia—are being researched to explore their possible connections to autoimmune function and later development of IBD.

Giardiasis is a microscopic bacteria found in water, and most likely comes from human waste. According to the Centers for Disease Control (CDC),

> "*Giardia* is a germ that causes diarrhea. *Giardia* is found in infected people's stool and cannot be seen by the naked eye. This germ is protected by an outer shell that allows it to survive outside the body and in the environment for long periods of time.
>
> During the past two decades, *Giardia* has become recognized as one of the most common causes of waterborne illness (drinking water and recreational water) in the United States. The germ is found in every part of the United States and the world."

Giardia is extremely contagious, and easily spread if proper hand washing is not performed. To get rid of the germ, I had to take a course of a strong antibiotic called Flagyl (metronidazole), which destroys *all* the flora and fauna in the gut. It wreaks havoc on the delicate balance and the chemical release in the gut, but most notably impacts the small intestine.

The treatment with Flagyl back in 1994 caused nausea, dizziness, and vomiting. It was a 5–10 day course and I was not made aware that I needed to follow up with any probiotic supplements (see page 39) to introduce "friendly" bacteria back into my digestive system.

Candida, a kind of yeast, can mimic many food particles that evoke an inflammatory response by the immune system cells located in the mucosal lining. This explains why many IBD patients can be especially sensitive to any yeast in their diet.

Dede's Experience

Many people, including one of my personal heroes, the Jacksonville Jaguars quarterback, David Garrard, have had great success taking medication to suppress the immune system and keep ulcerative colitis and Crohn's disease at bay.[7] While my husband and I learned everything we could after my initial diagnosis in 2001, drug therapy was daunting, and my disease at that time was moderate and not life-threatening. Again, using the Robert Frost metaphor, "the road less traveled" is sometimes the way to go (or not—each person makes their own, hopefully, informed choices).

When I read stories about athletes with Crohn's and colitis, I am so inspired. They represent a certain type of fighter, and Garrard, especially, has an inspiring story of overcoming disease, taking drugs, having surgery, and now balancing drug therapy (Remicade™) with a post-surgical outlook that is very promising. As of July, 2006, Garrard has been symptom-free. This past football season, he started a campaign with the CCFA called "In the Zone™ for Crohn's" to fight against Crohn's disease and ulcerative colitis. The foundation's mission is to find a cure for these painful and debilitating digestive diseases. To date, Garrard has raised $180,000 for the CCFA. To learn more about Garrard's amazing work, visit www.CrohnsintheZone. com.

Other athletes of recognition include Sam and Laura Kirstein; for both, IBD had halted their active lifestyles. I learned of their cross-country bicycle ride through the Mayo Clinic website and was impressed that they were able to ride 4,000 miles—in Sam's case post-surgery for ulcerative colitis!

There are numerous stories of athletes racing, walking, and biking with names like "Get Your Guts in Gear," and "Take Steps for Crohn's and Colitis," on the CCFA website.

This coming summer, on June 27th—which is a mere few days after the publication of this book—I am slated to run my first-ever half marathon in Boston to raise money for the CCFA's research. I have been inspired by other athletes who have gone before me, and I know I will be in good company with a group of IBD sufferers like myself.

THE POWER OF PROBIOTICS

Many microflora may prove beneficial in many *dysbiosis* states. Dysbiosis is the term we use to describe the imbalance that takes place when the gastrointestinal lining is not in homeostasis and therefore easily allows opportunistic infections to occur. In Crohn's disease, specifically, we note an aggressive T-lymphocyte mediated response to some, but not all, probiotics within the gastrointestinal tract lining. Appropriate and directed probiotic supplementation has shown to be beneficial in many studies and research also supports the idea that therapeutically manipulating microbial composition and function by antibiotics, probiotics, and/or prebiotics in an organized fashion could restore mucosal homeostasis in inflammatory bowel disease patients.[7]

MICROFLORA'S ROLE IN IBD AND MUCOSAL IMMUNE SYSTEM RELATION

One aspect of gastrointestinal health that is important to understand when discussing treatment options for Crohn's, UC, and other forms of IBD is *microbial balance*. Microbial balance is a term used to describe the ever-changing state of the beneficial *microorganisms* that live in our intestines. This mix of microorganisms such as probiotic bacteria and yeast make a significant contribution (and one which scientists are only just beginning to understand) to the health of the intestine and that of its host: the human body. One reason why the system of microorganisms is so hard to understand is that they are so huge in number; they outnumber our mammalian cells by at least ten fold.[8] In other words, *we are made up of significantly more bacteria than we are made up of our own cells.*

In a healthy human being, the *microorganisms* within the gastrointestinal tract, also referred to as *probiotics*, have many functions that contribute to the health of its host and provide a truly symbiotic relationship.

> Microflora, or probiotics, found in the gastrointestinal lining, are many but there are a few major players to note. Lactobacillus acidophilus, bifidobacterium, and saccharomyces cerevisiae (boulardii) are among the most common, but there are a multitude of others.

Microorganisms help increase proper enzyme activity within the intestine to facilitate proper breakdown of food and optimal absorption of nutrients. They also help to populate the intestinal lining to crowd out unhealthy microflora. But microorganisms play another important role: they help to establish a proper immune response. How? When in proper balance, microflora within the intestine stimulate the *mucosa cell immune system*. The mucosa cell immune system is a highly specialized part of the immune system made up of cells that comprise the mucosal lining and specific B- and T-lymphocytes. The mucosal lining acts as the very first line of defense regulating the passage of material in and out. The B- and T-lymphocytes work together in harmony to either stimulate the appropriate T-cell mediated and B-cell antibody related responses, or they come together to create systemic anergy (no reaction), also referred to as " oral tolerance," which was discussed earlier in this chapter.

With the help of microorganisms, the mucosa cell immune system functions just as it should. That is, not over-stimulating inflammatory cytokines, but not under-stimulating them either. Within the mucosa, there lies a need for a constant, minute amount of fluctuating inflammation. This inflammation serves to protect the organism and heal mucosa tissue.

There is now scientific evidence to support the action in which probiotic bacteria are able to penetrate the epithelial lining without causing a negative or inflammatory response that would normally be caused by other invading bacteria or viruses. This evidence suggests the truly symbiotic relationship we enjoy with the bacteria that inhabit our gastrointestinal mucosa. This is a good example of "oral tolerance". Our bodies are able to see the benefit probiotics offer us and, in turn, gives probiotic bacteria a special back stage pass to our mucosal immune system. There is also evidence that suggests inflammatory bowel disease may stem from a dysregulation of the responses to normal resident microflora within the mucosal immune system. Meaning that, in inflammatory bowel disease patients, the mucosal immune system is confused and begins mounting reactions against many antigens it's exposed to in addition to mounting reactions to the probiotic, symbiotic bacteria that would normally benefit them. Evidence of this lies in the fact that mice raised in completely sterile environments without the presence of microflora, even if they have a T-cell or B-cell dysfunction commonly related to inflammatory bowel disease, will still not exhibit the destructive inflammatory process normally seen in IBD sufferers. This evidence shows that possibly the first trigger of IBD is the improper reaction to probiotic bacteria. In the mice, the bacteria were not present and no symptoms of IBD were initiated.

In the near future, extensive research will be poured into finding probiotic bacteria that improve IBD patients. Current research in France has been underway in which scientists are studying a probiotic named *F. prausnitzii* to treat Crohn's patients and the results rendered a decrease in inflammation. This is promising because by using a specific probiotic, the body was able to build a symbiotic relationship and cease the initiation of inflammation.[9]

On a side note, there have been extensive studies done which support the connection of IBD and one's risk for thromboemboli, which is a blood clot (thrombus) that breaks loose and is carried by the blood stream to get stuck in another vessel. It is suggested that the connection between inflammatory bowel disease and risk for clotting is that endotoxins within the intestine interact with IL-1 and TNF-alpha and stimulate coagulation initiation.[10,11] This again stresses two things: the need for proper flora balance and probiotic supplementation and the need for lowering inflammation in IBD sufferers.

Again, a person's microbial balance will directly influence many aspects regarding their health including risks for certain diseases in addition to how they will respond to certain medical and lifestyle interventions.

Dede's Experience

My probiotic supplement is a powder that I mix daily in water with my ground Flax seed, and this is perhaps the most important act I do to keep myself in remission. As even natural herbal supplements can have adverse side effects, it is important to work with a naturopathic doctor, like Dr. Black, who has had the requisite four-year medical degree. I feel confident in taking herbal and mineral supplements, and they are of the purest quality. Although some may say that it's merely a placebo effect, I am convinced that I need the beneficial "live culture" bacteria added to my digestive tract. I am in my fourth year of full remission, and I am proud of this regimen and the obvious benefits to my overall health.

In addition to probiotics, prebiotics are natural plant compounds that help fuel beneficial intestinal bacteria, and these are recently being studied. There are classic treatment studies (involving the administration of a placebo, or a treatment, to test the efficacy of new medicines) that can be found on the CCFA website (ccfa. org), and there are broader non-therapeutic studies listed that involve following patients and relatives with IBD. I have had success calling the hospitals in my area to find out what studies are being done and requesting information on specific studies. Hospitals also administer their own data-driven studies, and I usually sign up for these so they can track my progress. It brings me hope, as a patient, to think that I can participate.

CHAPTER 4

Childhood Development and Gastrointestinal Disorders

INFLAMMATORY BOWEL disease usually affects individuals from ages 15 to 30, but can affect younger children as well. IBD in young children presents a unique challenge; oftentimes, younger children may maintain normal bowel function and exhibit no symptoms, and as a result damage and destruction can be occurring within the gastrointestinal tract months or years before diagnosis. Furthermore, diagnosis is more difficult in young children because their symptoms often resemble many other child and adolescent illnesses.

Diagnosis finally comes about because colon damage is progressive, and a young child will eventually begin showing symptoms of the disease. Once symptoms present themselves, further testing (such as such as X-rays, colonoscopies, and endoscopies) is required to confirm the diagnosis and look for bleeding and inflammation relating to the colon, stomach, esophagus, and small intestine.

Needless to say, the best way to help your child is to seek medical advice and attention as soon as they let you know they are experiencing repetitive gastrointestinal problems.

Dede's Experience

If you are a parent of an elementary-age child who suddenly starts complaining of tummy aches, it is important to remain calm and avoid acting alarmed, openly scared, or nervous because this can affect the child. In some cases, they may shy away from discussing stomach pain and/or diarrhea because these are embarrassing symptoms, so it is recommended that you try to keep open and honest communication with your child so that they can feel comfortable discussing his or her symptoms.

A great resource for parents and kids with IBD is this kid-centered site: http://kidshealth.org/parent/medical/digestive/ibd.html.

Another helpful resource is the CCFA-run Camp Oasis. After my surgery, I joined a support group through my hospital. A (then) ten-year-old girl in my group had real problems fitting in with her social group and refused to tell anyone, including her best friends, that she suffered from Crohn's disease. Her mother was at a loss about what to do with her during the summer, and I suggested Camp Oasis for her. I knew about this camp from the CCFA website and at the end of the summer, her mother reported back to me that the camp was the "best thing that has happened to her child" in many months, even years. It was a chance for this young person to be a kid again, to hang out with campers and counselors alike, who all suffered from the same debilitating disease, but didn't let it dampen their spirits or slow them down. All the normal activities, like swimming and just hanging out with other kids, were enjoyed and she has now gone back three years in a row! Other information is available on the CCFA website (ccfa.org), including planning for college and other resources.

TREATMENT

After your child is diagnosed, your doctor will determine the right course of treatment for your child's symptoms depending on the severity of illness. The initial treatment suggested in children with IBD usually includes an oral drug, such as sulfasalazine or mesalamine, which helps to reduce inflammation and stop flare ups. Suppositories can also be used initially if inflammation is great in the lower colon. Children who don't respond to these types of medication may be given a steroid drug like prednisone, though this is not ideal due to potential sides effects, especially if its use is needed long-term. As every case is different, it is vital that, when starting a supplement and dietary regimen, you seek the advice of a well-trained naturopathic physician or other practitioner.

Diet

The right diet is key to maintaining health. Some children will bounce back fairly quickly and inflammation can be kept under control rather easily, but it is important to stay loyal to the dietary suggestions and supplement routine. Even if a child gets well, if he stops all of his or her support, symptoms will likely return. Enforcing and maintaining the best diet is especially important for adolescents because they generally exhibit poor sleep and dietary habits. Parents should always remember that consistent lifestyle change and consistent support is vital for managing IBD symptoms in children and adolescents.

Most children will eat healthily if they are shown healthy eating habits by example. Drink water and your children will drink water. Eat vegetables, fruits, and whole grains (while not suitable for most sufferers, whole grains should be eaten if the individual does not have adverse reactions. Also see "Going off Wheat" on page 62) and your children will follow your example. Keep in mind, though, that children will undoubtedly go through their picky phases and also may go through mono-food stages, but they will generally pick up the habits of their parents. The best thing parents can do for their children's health is to follow healthy daily diet and lifestyle practices themselves.

Dede's Experience

As we've mentioned before, keeping a food journal is really important for sufferers of IBD, both young and old. A food journal is a great way for young IBD patients to feel more stable as it can also include anecdotes of the child's day, complete with pictures.

My food journal, after coming home from my bowel resection, began more as a note to my doctor that was somewhat humorous and sarcastic (for example, "Well, Dr. H, you *told* me to keep a food journal so here goes . . . this is going to be really boring since I now eat practically the same thing every day!"). Later on, as my food journal progressed, I began to explore how and why I started writing this book, and the so-called journal took on a life of its own.

A child's journal can include trips, playdates, or what the child ate. The journal can be a way to focus on the possibility of stressful situations and how to avoid them in the future, including which foods to avoid. It can also point out positive things such as safe foods or helpful and enjoyable experiences. Utilizing artwork such as drawings and collages in the child's journal are additional forms of expression that can be used to explore the positive and negative effects of disease on a child. Art therapy has been practiced for a long time, and for good reason. A journal can be private, but sharing and opening up to the specific impact of IBD on a child or teen is often very helpful. Both positive and negative entries should be encouraged. Any child (or adult, for that matter) who lives with IBD will have good days and bad days.

A well-balanced diet is key, and the suggestions in this book are vital, along with lifestyle support.

Monitoring diet and fluid intake is also important for keeping your child safe; in particular, it is important to look out for malnutrition in children and adolescents with IBD. Because of significant diarrhea resulting from the illness or reactions to medications they may be taking, nutrient loss may occur and can be life-threatening if not monitored appropriately. Sometimes vitamin supplements may be required. Anemia and low vitamin D levels are also prevalent among children with inflammatory bowel disease.[1] Supplementation with vitamin D, B vitamins, and iron can help reduce long-term illness of IBD patients.

Dede's Experience

Children and teens are unfortunately a fast-growing segment of the Crohn's and ulcerative colitis community.

For children and teens with Crohn's, it is even harder to do things like go to school, attend parties, or eat the same food the other kids are eating. While the joy of attending Camp Oasis has been well-documented, every child will not have the opportunity to go to camp each summer. Keeping a food journal with your child is a great way to get them involved, as is joining a support group, and talking with teachers, camp counselors and family members to help your child or teen cope and navigate the difficulties of living with an incurable disease. Children and teens have unique concerns and may need additional support to address issues like anorexia and stunted growth. In a child's mind, if eating makes them sick, why would they want to eat? Hence, issues such as anorexia and malnutrition may arise. A great deal of support is needed during the diagnostic stage, and later on during the treatment stages.

Many tests, like barium enemas used to assess intestinal blockages, are highly invasive and painful. Luckily, IBD clinics nationwide are beginning to conform to the specific needs of their youngest IBD patients, which will help ease the process for them.

Treatment with Medications

Due to elevated C-reactive protein levels and elevated erythrocyte sedimentation rates, which are two ways to evaluate inflammation in the body, many children benefit from anti-inflammatory medication. Immunosuppressive drugs are also used in some children, adolescents, and adults for a period of time, but should be considered as absolute last drugs of choice because of the risks involved with long-term use. When using immunosuppressive drugs, such as TNF-α inhibitors, the longer an individual takes them, the higher their risk for other chronic illnesses such as cancer, which is normally kept under control by the regulatory effects of the immune system.

CHILDHOOD GUT HEALTH AND ITS AFFECT ON INFLAMMATORY BOWEL DISEASE

Preliminary influences on the gastrointestinal tract and immune system can mold future genetic expression for disease. Oftentimes, these influences occur even before the child is born.

In the womb, the fetus is not exposed to any microflora. A baby begins generating its massive microbial milieu the minute it passes through the vaginal canal. Cesarean section babies do not acquire a proper balance of flora early in infancy, therefore supplementing C-section babies for the first 6 months of life with probiotics appropriate to infants can help to ward off allergy and disease potential.[2] Bifidobacterium becomes the predominant probiotic to supplement infants at least until 12 months of age. The proper balance of probiotics we begin with as infants becomes extremely important in the potential of developing IBD due to the strong connection between microbial problems, inflammation, and IBD.

PROMOTING HEALTHY CHILDHOOD DEVELOPMENT

True prevention of chronic illness is attained through the preservation of optimal childhood health and development.

The infant's or child's body must be supported and enhanced in order to learn and develop proper responses to illnesses. The physiology of a child's body is very sensitive and will alter its functions based on its total environment, inside and out. Promoting this proper childhood development is the cornerstone to preventing future health issues! Proper diet, a supportive emotional environment within the home, proper lifestyle modeling from parents, and effective daily routines to help maintain optimal glandular and elimination organ function are only a few aspects of an advantageous chronic disease prevention program.

Acidophilus

Often times in infancy and childhood, taking an acidophilus supplement can serve as an effective tool in helping the mucosal immune system develop. As the mucosal immune system develops it can, in turn, help the body's overall immune system generate its own balance in its reactions and in regard to what it should consider safe. Acidophilus has also been shown to reduce the incidence of allergies and prevent long durations of acute illnesses.

As stated earlier, C-section babies acquire at birth a completely different subset of microorganisms to inhabit their gastrointestinal tracts. Acidophilus supplements given to C-section babies reduce allergy risk in the future. This information becomes much more important than merely decreasing allergy risk, and it extends to decreased autoimmune disease, cancer risk, and chronic illness risk compared to other C-section babies who were not replenished with corrective probiotic strains of bacteria.

EMOTIONS AND IBD

Like an innate need, the extremely personal and intimate communication between a baby and a caregiver stimulates the baby's central nervous system and the part of their brain called the limbic brain, which is responsible for developing memories and storing emotions. If babies do not get this interchange, they can become irritable, uncomfortable, and under developed.[3] This can skew the body's balanced responses, including balance within the gastrointestinal border. At the same time, if a child has the genetic tendency for IBD but has been raised in the appropriate health supporting environment in development, he or she will have a reduced chance of developing IBD compared with children whose environments are not conducive to a healing and balanced immune response.

One perfect example of immune system function being affected by childhood environment discussed that childhood maltreatment resulted in elevated inflammation levels in adults. Published in the

Archives of General Psychiatry, the study found that emotional distraction, neglect, and early emotional stress in children resulted in impaired immune function. Specifically, physical abuse in children was directly related to impaired immune system function, depression, and inflammation in adulthood.[4]

Dede's Experience

No-Talk Therapy for Children and Adolescents, by Dr. Martha B. Straus is an innovative approach to treatment of young clients who won't or can't respond to conversation-based therapy, and it might be worth looking into.

In the case of children with IBD or other autoimmune diseases, their development may be hindered both physically and emotionally. Their language and playing skills may be delayed or inhibited, making diagnosis and therapeutic help more challenging.

Straus provides many examples in her book that highlight children who do not work well with traditional therapies because, for obvious reasons, their young lives have been fraught with obstacles that even adults could find difficult. When I give talks about living with inflammatory bowel disease, I always try to address the concerns of younger members in the audience or support group: they are perhaps the most challenged in terms of adjusting to life on medication or post-surgery. Developing self-confidence after a diagnosis of IBD can be a challenge for a child and a concern for parents or caregivers. When I read the case histories in Straus's well-written book, I immediately thought of many young children with Crohn's disease or UC and their inability to express their emotions verbally. By giving children and teens a voice of their own, therapists can offer a safe place for those dealing with the pitfalls and struggles of living with IBD.

VACCINATIONS AND SUPPRESSIVE CARE IN EARLY LIFE

In a growing human being, allowing the immune system to develop properly is the key to lifelong health. Studies have shown that children's immune systems don't fully mature until about 6 or 7 years of age and their gastrointestinal tracts and livers are not fully developed until the age of 4.[5] Awareness of this growth and allowing the immune system to develop properly in the child is important for every parent.

Throughout childhood, a child's immune system develops and establishes how the body will defend itself from disease. Every bacteria, virus, and foreign antigen exposed to the body gives it practice for developing appropriate immune responses. Supportive care (for example, probiotic supplementation, proper food introduction, and avoiding suppressive treatments such as antibiotics and Tylenol) of the mucosal immune system in early developing years becomes extremely important in immune response later on. It helps to form the protective mucosal barrier that is so important for IBD patients. Allowing the immune system to become stronger through exposure to a variety of illnesses is key to guarding future health. Treatments that dampen the immune system through childhood and adolescence, called suppressive treatments (including, but not limited to, antibiotics, Tylenol, and reflux medications), may damper the immunological reaction so that the immune system cannot exercise its ability to respond to infections.

Our body's response to infection is perfectly orchestrated toward healing. For example, the body mounts a fever for a reason: during an infection, the body uses a fever as an immune response. The increase in temperature speeds up enzyme reactions and antibody production, and this allows healing or repair to occur more optimally. This system must be carefully guarded in a child whose immune system is still developing. For children, taking Tylenol during a fever can suppress this naturally occurring immune response, making the body less efficient at fighting the infection while prolonging sickness. Thus, the Mayo Clinic website suggests not giving a child Tylenol during fever unless the fever is over 101°F. In the case when a child has a fever under 101°F and Tylenol is not being given, constitutional hydrotherapy treatments given at home can be extremely effective for reducing fevers and helping children feel better, sleep easier, and recover more quickly.

Vaccinations can also pose problems in relationship to a child's developing immunity.

Introducing virus and bacteria combinations and other foreign antigens can be risky for infants and children who lack mature immune systems and organ function.

If the small infant body is just beginning to work on generating immune tolerance, or oral tolerance as described earlier, it is very likely that simultaneously introducing many foreign antigens directly into the blood stream will cause confusion within the immune system. In the general population, most people understand the importance of waiting to introduce foods to infants slowly to avoid creating allergies and allow the infant to develop increased oral tolerance slowly and naturally. Yet it isn't considered that injecting significant amounts of foreign material into the blood stream may affect immunuological response in addition to future immune balance, health, and disease risk.

Antibiotics give rise to further concern. Because in recent years they have been overused and abused, an unfortunate number of the population has become sensitive to them and bacteria have become antibiotic resistant. Antibiotic resistance is the ability of bacteria or other microbes to resist the effects of an antibiotic treatment. Here is an excerpt from the CDC's website:

> "Antibiotic use promotes development of antibiotic-resistant bacteria. Every time a person takes antibiotics, sensitive bacteria are killed, but resistant germs may be left to grow and multiply. Repeated and improper uses of

antibiotics are primary causes of the increase in drug-resistant bacteria.

While antibiotics should be used to treat bacterial infections, they are not effective against viral infections like the common cold, most sore throats, and the flu. Widespread use of antibiotics promotes the spread of antibiotic resistance. Smart use of antibiotics is the key to controlling the spread of resistance."[6]

The sensitive bacteria the CDC refers to are probiotics. Each time a child takes antibiotics, it potentially kills off the bad bacteria, but also kills off the good bacteria, which can leave them more susceptible to future infections. If antibiotics are used, they should be used extremely rarely and always followed by aggressive probiotic therapy of long duration in order to re-build the mucosal immune defense.

Antibiotics and IBD

Overuse of antibiotics prior to or after diagnosis of IBD can significantly affect one's prognosis of the disease. Overuse of antibiotics kills off a significant proportion of good probiotic bacteria, leaving an individual vulnerable to the next microbial invasion by removing part of the important mucosal barrier to infection. Disrupting this border affects reactions to foods, inflammation, and can worsen IBD symptoms. According to Dr. Ronald Hoffman, founder and Medical Director of the Hoffman Center in New York City and author of numerous health books, the epidemic-like spread of Crohn's disease over roughly the last 50 years started with the introduction of antibiotics and developed in parallel with an increase in antibiotic consumption. Find physicians in your area that are comfortable in treating children without the use of antibiotics. If antibiotics are used, they should be used extremely rarely and always followed by aggressive probiotic therapy of long duration in order to re-build the mucosal immune defense.

A PARENT'S ROLE IN THE HEALING PROCESS

It can be extremely frustrating and exhausting to have an ill child. Our hope is that this book can guide you in helping your child attain improved wellness. Many of the suggestions in this book are focused on adults but many are appropriate for children and teenagers.

> Teenagers who weigh close to an adult weight can do and take most of the treatments. Before implementing any hormone programs such as DHEA, we suggest you seek medical advice.

Dede's Experience

In her groundbreaking book, *Breaking the Vicious Cycle*, Elaine Gottshall's child was diagnosed with severe ulcerative colitis and, as a mother, she had no choice but to search everywhere for a cure, which was achieved through adherence to a strict carbohydrate-free diet.

Some sections in her book really helped me; for example, she explains that table sugar is a trisaccharide whereas honey is a monosaccharide, thereby easier for the body to break down. Since I don't have a biochemical degree, I always felt intimidated about understanding food and ingredients, but this book has served me well and helps me in eating a simple, easy-to-digest diet.

After my diagnosis in 2001, I tried to follow the dietary guidelines in Gottshall's book. However, I had trouble sticking to it at that time because it is very rigid. Nowadays, with the rise of inflammatory bowel disease and other autoimmune diseases like rheumatoid arthritis and celiac disease, Gottshall's is a very pertinent and important book, and the diet guidelines are a bit easier to follow now that stores nationwide and overseas are carrying many products that are wheat- and dairy-free.

Herbal teas are extremely beneficial for children and can provide profound effects if used consistently. There is no maximum dosage for teas in children. Herbal formulas, drainage remedies, homeopathic remedies, and even enemas can all be used safely on children if used correctly. Specific vitamins and supplements may have dosage alterations to accommodate children. A good way to determine how much your child can handle is to determine how their weight relates to an average adult. For example, if they weigh 50 lbs., most likely they can tolerate ⅓ of the dosage an adult can take, assuming the average adult is 150 lbs. Usually this rule can help you find a starting dosage for your child. Children can typically take nearly half the adult dose as soon as they reach 50 lbs. You can also research to see if a particular supplement has any toxicity or maximum dosage for children.

Dietary changes almost always help children very quickly with symptoms. The stricter you are with the dietary changes, the more likely you will see change. In children, it is especially helpful to take out dairy, sugar, processed foods, and sometimes all gluten.

HOPE FOR A HEALTHY FUTURE

The beautiful thing about children is they have so much more vitality than adults and will respond fairly quickly to treatment. Due to their increased vitality, children have a larger potential for becoming and remaining symptom-free through life if they continue with the dietary, lifestyle, and supplement support that helped them improve in the first place.

Remember that children with IBD or any illness will need constant emotional support while growing up because it is hard to be different. Tender loving care and emotional availability as a parent is vital to the healing process.

CHAPTER 5

Musculoskeletal and Diet-Related Causes of Inflammatory Bowel Disease

A S STATED earlier, there is not yet a known cure for IBD. However, there is still hope for those with the condition: research has shown that proper diet can help to relieve symptoms and increase the effectiveness of many treatments. Those afflicted can take an active role in guarding their health and improving their lives. Knowing how to eat well is the first step.

In his book *The New Eating Right for a Bad Gut,* Dr. James Scala explains,

"As of now, nothing can cure IBD, including all modern drugs, herbs, nostrums, devices, and surgery! Diet can reduce the symptoms and flare-ups and make them less severe. Most important, it can help reduce medication by a large measure, or shift control to a milder drug. Many people will be able to stop taking daily medication and require a less potent drug if a flare-up occurs, which is reason enough to follow the diet. Surgery often, but not always, stops the progression of IBD, even if the patient has to live with a pouch or colostomy, and the diet is helpful for people even after surgery."[1]

It is extremely important that IBD sufferers pay close attention to what they eat and have a working knowledge of which foods are good for them and which they should avoid.

HOW DO FOODS STIMULATE INFLAMMATION?

The first step to learning how to eat well is to understand how poor food choices can worsen IBD.

Foods that commonly cause reactions in individuals suffering from inflammatory conditions are the following:

- Wheat and sometimes even gluten which is a constituent of wheat and other grains such as barley and spelt
- Dairy
- Sugar
- Potatoes
- Tomatoes
- Eggplant
- Peppers
- Paprika
- Cayenne
- Tobacco

Dede's Experience: Going Off Wheat

People always ask me why I can't eat wheat, and I don't have a clear answer. I remember my naturopath asking me to give up wheat when I was having digestive issues—mostly constipation and blockages—and I was horrified. "I love pizza and bagels the most," I pleaded with her. She demured and suggested I give up wheat for three days to see if that helped my frequent bouts of arthritis (a result of long-term flares of Crohn's disease that ravaged my joints).

After three days, I was ecstatic. I had more energy, and I felt better all over, especially in my elbows and knees which were frequently arthritic. Four years have now passed, and I switched to the ancient wheat grain, Spelt, for my occasional wheat-fixes (though I typically use rice flour for pastas and pizza crusts). Spelt looks very similar to wheat—just ask my seventeen-year-old son who often samples my Spelt concoctions, like pizza dough and scones, and doesn't notice any difference from the same made with wheat! Spelt actually contains more protein than wheat, and since I eat very little red meat, I do like getting extra protein in my diet. In addition, the protein is easier to digest; however, there is actually more gluten in Spelt, which makes it an unsuitable grain for those with celiac disease.

As far as oats are concerned, I have found this grain to be easier to digest than most other whole grains. According to nutritionist and food specialist at the University of Vermont Diane Lamb in her excellent column in the Brattleboro *Reformer*,

> "Breakfast can make your day! . . . A healthy breakfast should energize you, satisfy your hunger and provide beneficial nutrients—carbohydrates, protein, vitamins, minerals, and a small amount of fat . . . A bowl of cereal (hot or cold) that has some dietary fiber with low-fat milk or yogurt, fruit, and even a few nuts provides a lot more nutrients than an empty calorie food like that sweet roll, or donut. . . . In addition to lowering blood cholesterol, oats (oatmeal) can help control blood sugar and insulin sensitivity. Whole grains including oatmeal are digested more slowly than refined grains. This

slower digestion leads to a gradual, steady supply
of blood sugar which can keep hunger in check."

I rely heavily on routine in my diet and lifestyle choices.
I always read labels carefully, and I try to cook with
McCann's Steel Cut oats, perhaps as a nod to my Irish
heritage, but more importantly, to get the purest grain
without any addition of refined sugars, added salt, and
flavors. Sometimes the fewer ingredients on the label, the
happier I am and more apt to purchase!

As all individuals are different, even within the same disease personal reactions can vary considerably. For example, Jane may react
to oranges and wheat and have rectal bleeding, and Peter may react
severely to eggplant and tomato with the symptom of diarrhea. Other
foods to be aware of for reactions are corn, white rice, dried fruit,
citrus fruits, ALL processed comfort foods, pastries, cookies, desserts, etc. Many IBD patients have a hard time with this because they
have eaten these foods for a long time and have started experiencing
bowel problems. What you must understand is that when we list all
of the potential causes of illness, we are referring to one's total load,
or total capacity to take things in and still remain in good health.

Dede's Experience:

Smoking and Crohn's Disease

Crohn's disease can perhaps be triggered in a genetically
susceptible person or perhaps by an infection. Maybe
something unknown triggers an immune alarm that sets
off a digestive tract inflammation. Since there is no

documented cause of the disease, Crohn's disease sufferers are frequently in limbo about which type of drug or treatment to pursue while working toward a normal life.

For many, smoking may not cause the disease but can certainly aggravate symptoms. I spoke to my doctors, Jeffry Potash and Steven Bensen, about my smoking history, and they were interested to learn that I had smoked for almost 20 years prior to the onset of Crohn's disease. I remember telling them that smoking almost seemed like "a diuretic" for me, and that may have been the case. In fact the opposite was more likely happening. Smoking affects the entire body in a negative way; in particular, the intestines are affected by a lack of blood flow to the area caused by nicotine and a rise in acid in the stomach—which, in turn, affects the lining of the intestines. Because this has been documented, Crohn's disease and UC patients are encouraged to quit smoking.

Those patients who have Crohn's disease are more affected by nicotine than those with ulcerative colitis—a number of studies report that Crohn's patients who smoked had a higher incidence of inflammation and scarring in the terminal ileum than other areas of the intestine (as in my case).

I grew up with two parents who smoked. It has been well documented that smoking is addictive and harmful to the heart and lungs; now we can look specifically to Crohn's disease and see a link to nicotine. Just as exercise can help to alleviate some of the symptoms of Crohn's disease, cessation of smoking can alleviate the symptoms as well. Interestingly, in some patients with UC, their symptoms have been documented to lessen when they inhale nicotine and restrict the blood flow to the colon.

My struggle to quit smoking lasted quite a while. For a period of around 3 years, I tried hypnosis, acupuncture, and nicotine patches—all to no avail. Finally, I tried hypnosis one more time, and that seemed to get me on the right track. It was very expensive to undergo hypnosis, but many hospitals offer free smoking cessation classes. In fact, there are many such support groups available. During those first (crucial to success) three weeks of my plan, I would often treat myself to fruit juice smoothies at our local food co-op. These drinks were rather expensive ($3–4 each); however, I justified the expense since I wasn't spending money on outrageously expensive packs of cigarettes. When my cravings got severe, I would rush to the store and buy a smoothie.

My smoothie recipe is as follows:
- ½ cup frozen strawberries (organic)
- ½ cup frozen blueberries (organic, and I usually freeze in the summertime after I pick)
- 1 cup non-fat yogurt
- ½ cup 1% lowfat milk
- 2 tablespoons of maple syrup.

Put all in the blender and mix. Serves 1–2.

When you are craving something sweet, choose unrefined sugar or natural sweeteners. They contain small amounts of nutrients so they won't deplete your system as much as refined sugar does.

ALLERGENS

One of the biggest problems present in food is allergens. *Allergens* stimulate a response from the immune system. Allergens in foods can occur naturally, or they can be the result of additives or preservatives added to the foods.

As mentioned earlier, oral tolerance develops as infants when foods are introduced to our gastrointestinal tract for the first time. Most of the time, our bodies make an important decision to allow foods into the gastrointestinal tract without mounting defensive immune reactions; this is important so that foods can be broken down into nutrients to be used by the body for energy. If oral tolerance develops incorrectly due to circumstances such as environment, genetics, or improper food introduction, allergies can result.

Interestingly, food allergies most often are associated with low stomach acid also called hydrochloric acid. To understand why, it's important to have a basic understanding of digestion. Digestion is dependant on a three step process.

The first step, called pre-digestion, occurs within the mouth and esophagus; the second is a period of further breakdown via stomach acid and pepsin in the stomach. The third step involves further breakdown with digestive enzymes in the small intestine where nutrient absorption finally occurs.

The digestion process can be affected during all three of these steps in digestive illnesses. The first step of the process, the pre-digestion of foods in the mouth and esophagus, can be affected by the foods we choose. Low enzyme content or processed and packaged foods lead to less pre-digestion and more undigested foods and proteins in the stomach. Over time, this takes a toll on how much acid our bodies can produce. In addition to increased aging, this excess stress on digestion in the stomach can cause reduced stomach acid levels.

The third process of digestion can be affected by lack of pancreatic digestive enzymes leading to compromised digestion of food particles. Less effective digestion, no matter what the cause, simply means larger food particles and proteins in the blood stream. Larger proteins in the blood stream lead to immune response and food allergies.

Another effect can also occur when individuals with low stomach acid consume food. The small amount of stomach acid they have is not enough to completely digest the meal, and larger food particles are left over. These undigested foods can cause fermentation to occur within the bowel. The fermentation manifests itself with symptoms such as gas, bloating, and upset stomach. Fermenting and undigested food provokes a response from the immune system, usually resulting in increased inflammation through rising histamine levels. This also supports the connection between reactions to foods and allergic responses triggered by the immune system. As explained earlier, anti-histamines reduce allergy symptoms because they reduce histamine, which is the compound responsible for increasing allergy symptoms. Magnesium is needed to reduce histamine levels as well, so make sure to supplement with magnesium for any allergy issues.[2] In fact, magnesium is often the first supplement of choice for many IBD patients, assuming they don't have diarrhea. See more about magnesium in the treatment section.

Low stomach acid levels not only cause issues with allergies, it also reduces levels of beneficial intestinal bacteria, which are needed for absorption of magnesium. This creates a vicious cycle. When acid levels are too low, this causes lower absorption capability for magnesium; as a result, depressed magnesium levels can't help keep histamine levels under control. Higher histamine levels increase inflammation and increase allergy symptoms.

What is in Our Food?

There are more than a few reasons why so many people are experiencing rising inflammation from eating certain foods coupled with food intolerances and allergies. People are reacting to the innate nature of the food and its chemical structure. In addition, due to high-stress lifestyles, lack of live-enzyme content of our food and general aging, low stomach acid is nearly inevitable in most people. In the next chapter, we will discuss the connection between stress and cortisol levels, and how these factors lead to low stomach acid. This low stomach acid and resulting fermentation in the stomach adds to inflammation levels and illness. Currently there are so many food additives in most foods that people consume, that the additives themselves pose significant risk for increasing inflammation and provoking allergenic or intolerant-type reactions.

There are a number of additives and chemicals found in our foods that can affect health. Pesticide residues are not the only compounds found in food. There are heavy metals found in some fish, there are preservatives, coloring chemicals, additives for flavors, man-made fats, industrial waste chemicals, and so on. Many of these unnecessary chemicals pose potential harm to the immune system. Most of these chemicals, due to their irritant nature, can stimulate inflammatory processes within the body.

Take MSG, for example. It is an additive that works as a flavor enhancer that is used in many foods and has a strong reputation for provoking allergy responses in people. Many Crohn's patients are unable to tolerate MSG. Food dyes are known to increase asthma attacks and exacerbate ADD and ADHD symptoms. Pesticide residues have been linked to cancers,[3] neurological conditions,[4] and so on.

Dede's Experience

When I first started keeping a food journal, I discovered very quickly that I would need to avoid MSG after having eaten a take-out dinner from a local Chinese restaurant, which was followed by cramps and a mild flare-up. After that, I have always requested a non-MSG dinner.

Another food I noted in my food journal as causing cramping was corn on the cob. I remember thinking it would be safe to put the corn in a blender and puree it so that it could be digested easily (similar to baby food). However, this only caused me to have a flare-up of Crohn's disease quicker than if I had eaten kernels of corn! Corn is known for traveling through the digestive system very quickly—parents of young children know this when they change a diaper that even has intact kernels in the soiled diaper—so it is important to chew the kernels very well in your mouth to start the process of digestion. I found that I could ingest corn tortillas easily, but it was the kernel that was problematic for me. Everyone—whether they are young, old, with Crohn's, UC or celiac disease—is different, with a unique set of digestive concerns.

MUSCULOSKELETAL CAUSES

Although it may not seem obvious, physical trauma to the body (musculoskeletal causes) can lead to IBD. Musculoskeletal stressors are important to address because even minor falls or injuries can have a negative impact on the proper functioning of the nervous system. The nervous system guides and directs the functioning of every organ in the body, including the intestines. Nerves signal when to speak, when to move, how to sense pain, how to digest foods, how to taste food, how to eliminate properly through our elimination organs, how to feel emotion, and so on. If our nervous system, the director, isn't working properly, then we have compromised systemic functioning. This applies to every part of the body; can you imagine if the nerve input to your bowels was inhibited or altered? Nutrient absorption and bowel elimination would be directly affected.

Dede's Experience

Integrative Manual Therapy is an effective treatment modality that assesses and treats pain and disease using the spinal cord to move the body's energy around.

Developed by Sharon Giammatteo, Ph.D., I.M.T.C., and colleagues over the past 30 years, IMT is a hands on technique that uses a gentle manipulation for fascial connective tissue repair (fascia is a sheet of connective tissue covering or binding together body structures). When injury or trauma occurs in the body, there is structural damage that is usually treated with first aid and follow-up physical therapy. With IMT, a balanced repair of surrounding tissue is also attempted in order to achieve rehabilitation. Once the structural integrity is restored, the function of the muscle or joint, or perhaps even the organ, can be affected for longer-lasting health benefits.

My good friend whom I consider a healer, Deborah Feiner-Homer, is my therapist in this hands-on technique. Years ago, I went to see Deborah for physical therapy after one of my knee surgeries. Although I was initially skeptical of her work in IMT, after my bowel resection I am now a convert to this kind of cranial sacral therapy.

This is ground-breaking work as far as I am concerned! I lie on her table and listen to her soothing voice as she lays one of her hands on my abdomen, and the other underneath my backside. I relax, and sometimes even cry in relief as I feel my pain subsiding . . . this coming from the stoic, uptight, "type A" professional woman I thought I was!

Think of how the body is affected during a spinal cord injury when complete nerve input is cut off from the rest of the body. When someone has a spinal cord injury, they may completely lose function of some organs but maintain partial function of others depending on where the nerves or injury is located. Now imagine an injury that stresses that same area in the spinal cord but does not sever the spinal cord. This injury stresses the nerve response back and forth from the brain to organs—but it may go undetected for years because the function still occurs at suboptimal levels. This is why injuries, even injuries from your past, should be reviewed and treated if necessary to ensure proper and timely healing.

TAKING RESPONSIBILITY FOR OUR BODIES

Our bodies were meant to be cherished, not ignored or taken for granted. Our bodies are our vehicles of our environment. We use our bodies to survive, communicate, eat, sleep, and exist. We must understand the significant impact of diet, lifestyle, and injury on our bodies' functions. Proper digestion, proper nutrient absorption from a healthy diet, and proper nerve function results in a healthier body—and a healthier body promotes a healthier, happier, and sounder mind.

CHAPTER 6

The Importance of
Balance in the Body

E VERY MOMENT, our bodies are constantly working to maintain balance, whether it be through proper hormone levels, or the synchronization of our various organs and organ systems. This natural balance within our bodies is impacted by many factors, including genetic risk, social stresses, environment, and diet (for example, chemicals found in our foods as discussed in the previous chapter).

When these factors become significant enough to disrupt our body's balance, disease can occur. Inflammatory bowel disease, in particular, is greatly influenced by disruptions in the body's natural balances.

HOW IMBALANCE CAN CAUSE DISEASE

To better understand how the body's homeostasis can influence the onset or severity of IBD, picture an 8 oz. cup. The contents of this cup look different for each person and is filled with everything they have been exposed to in their lifetime, including genetically inherited disease potential, genetically inherited toxicity, viruses, bacteria, physical stress, emotional stress, poor diet, sedentary lifestyle, injuries or accidents that inhibit or affect nervous system function, and so on. For many IBD patients, these factors greatly influence the way their bodies respond to certain foods. The more one has in their cup at a particular time, the less they are able to ingest allergenic foods without a negative response.

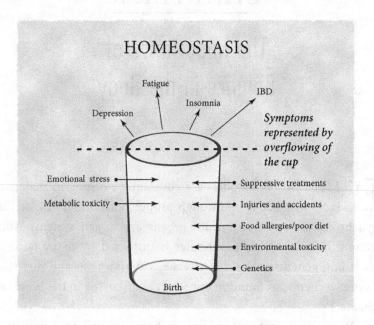

In each person, as this cup fills up with these factors for internal imbalance, there may come a breaking point at which the internal environment is so overwhelmed that it will result in symptoms. We will relate this breaking point to the overflowing of the cup.

If then the person goes to a doctor and is only treated for their symptoms, it is similar to putting a lid on the cup—combating the symptoms alone may be effective momentarily, but what happens when the treatment is either discontinued, or worse, stops working? Then the cup overflows again and symptoms return.

MAINTAINING THE RIGHT APPROACH IN TREATING IBD

The initial treatments for all illness, including IBD, should begin by addressing what caused the symptoms in the first place—an imbalance in the body. In the case of IBD, this would involve increasing proper function of all elimination organs (including the kidney, liver, and gastrointestinal tract). We refer to these elimination organs as *emunctory organs*. As the function of emunctory organs improve, we see great improvements in health. That being said, as people get well and treatments are geared towards their internal environment, the hope is that they are able to tolerate more foods without eruption of symptoms, but they should still not fall back into poor dietary and lifestyle habits.

It is important to remember that creating and maintaining wellness takes time and commitment. If one uses treatments and changes lifestyle habits until symptoms stop, but then they resume the habits that created the problem in the first place, the symptoms will return. When under treatment for chronic illness, it is important to realize that treatment beyond the cessation of symptoms is vital to health and maintaining disease remission.

WHAT DO HORMONES DO?

In order to better understand how our body's internal balance impacts IBD, it is important to also discuss hormones within the body. Hormones are chemical messengers made and used by the body to drive metabolic reactions. When we think of hormones, we tend to only think of estrogen, progesterone, and testosterone, which happen to be our sex hormones involved in many related processes including hair growth, sex drive, menstruation, fertility, aggression, energy, and more. But in addition to these common hormones, there are many other hormones used by the body to drive all body processes. Hormones influence our sleep, moods, immune reactions, blood pressure, blood sugar, energy, metabolism, etc.

The rate of biosynthesis of hormones is regulated by a negative feedback homeostatic mechanism. This means that if there is an excess amount of a particular hormone in circulation, it will provide negative feedback to where it was secreted from to prevent more of this hormone from being secreted. Similarly, if there is not enough of one hormone present, a positive feedback will be sent to stimulate more production and secretion of the needed hormone. In this way, our body maintains balanced levels of hormones in order to allow for proper functioning of our many internal processes.

When hormones are out of balance, we often see irritability, depression, insomnia, fatigue, and many other mental-emotional disorders. Hormone imbalances can also bring about, or exacerbate, symptoms in IBD patients. The entire immune response is driven by hormone regulation and balance. In turn, the hormones secreted by the immune system target specific tissues and stimulate the release of specific immune cytokines, which can result in inflammation in the GI tract and IBD if the hormones are not in balance.

In Chapter 8, we will discuss some options for IBD patients in controlling hormone balance, thus reducing some symptoms.

INTERCONNECTED ORGAN FUNCTION

When looking at gastrointestinal or other illnesses, it is also important to understand the connections between organs within the body.

Every organ in the body depends on, and influences, other organs—everything is interconnected in the body. This is why whole body approaches to healing often work better than treating just one system, or one symptom.

The gastrointestinal tract is a great example of how a single organ can influence, and be influenced by, many other organs within the body, and how any disruption in these connections can impact diseases such as IBD.

The gastrointestinal tract and the liver depend upon each other for optimal functioning. The liver has many functions, including making and breaking down hormones, detoxification, breaking down red blood cells, storing glycogen, metabolizing cholesterol, and maintaining general metabolism. The liver also makes bile, which is stored in the gallbladder and secreted into the small intestine to aid digestion of fats. Because the liver supports the production of hormones, it also plays a part in the production of cytokines that balance inflammation in the gastrointestinal tract.

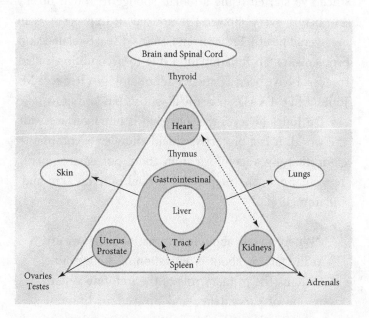

The liver, gastrointestinal tract, and how they are related to our organs.

According to Chinese medicine, the spleen is another key organ involved in gastrointestinal disorders. The spleen's main responsibilities are transforming and transporting food in the body, including the excretion of waste material. The spleen is also a major immune system organ, making it influential in the process of digestion and the inflammation present in IBD.

The two main outlets for the gastrointestinal tract are the lungs and the skin. If there are imbalances or stresses occurring within the gastrointestinal tract, this can directly impact the functioning of the lungs and the skin. For example, the skin can get worse initially when treatment for IBD begins, but will then improve over time when the gastrointestinal tract is healthier.

Dede's Experience

Since I've started using a loofah sponge to rough up my skin before every shower, I've noticed an improvement in my overall health. Either from Crohn's disease-related skin problems, or an inflammation due to a condition called rosacea, I have been a patient of dermatologist Rebecca M. Jones, M.D., FAAD, since my diagnosis ten years ago.

Dr. Jones believes that our skin is our interface with the world. It is a protective shield and also a 'communicator' that gives us information about our environment. For our book, she prepared a special note on skin and inflammation:

"When we talk about inflammation, what we are really talking about is activation of the immune system. The primary role of the immune system is one of surveillance and protection. Immune cells are charged with fighting off invaders, be they parasites, bacteria, viruses or even cancers. It makes sense, then, that the immune system is lined up like a military phalanx anywhere that our body faces the outside world. The skin is an obvious example of such an interface, but the gut and the lungs are also exposed to the environment, through anything we breathe and eat.

The skin, respiratory system and gastrointestinal system are all possible entry sites for infection. If we consider the harsh pressures that humans were up against before the invention of such things as antibiotics and sanitation, it makes sense that our immune system 'erred on the side of caution'. That is, the immune system might sometimes overreact, but evolutionarily this was better than underreacting and letting a parasite or bacteria invade and kill us.

There is reason to believe that many of our inflammatory disorders—ulcerative colitis, Crohn's disease, but also asthma, eczema and Psoriasis—represent the immune system's well intentioned, but mistaken, efforts to fight off what it thinks are parasites or bacteria—that is, the immune system overreacts. Very often the actual trigger isn't at all clear. For instance, most inflammatory disorders are easily triggered by stress."

THE HEART

The heart is the master of the body and emperor of all organs, including the gastrointestinal tract. According to traditional Chinese medicine, one of the oldest and most utilized medical models in the world, the heart's relationship to the body is hierarchical, meaning it governs and guides all internal functions of the body. If the heart is not balanced, circulation and rhythmic guiding of gastrointestinal function and digestion will be disrupted and disease can result.

The adrenals are also connected with the gastrointestinal tract because they secrete cortisol, which directly influences inflammatory disease states, such as IBD. In times of excess cortisol, the immune system is typically suppressed, which keeps the inflammation down. This explains why prednisone, which mimics cortisone and suppresses the immune response, helps in inflammatory bowel disease and many other inflammation-related illnesses. However, while an individual who has IBD is on prednisone, they may enjoy a lessening of their symptoms, but not without cost. If the entire immune system is suppressed by the prednisone, defense against foreign organisms is also decreased, along with immunological repair. These subtle changes exemplify the importance of maintaining balance within the body and can eventually cause larger problems if prednisone is used for long periods of time.

Dede's Experience

I've often wondered where expressions like "I feel it in my gut," or the ubiquitous "butterflies in my stomach," came from. As a layperson, writer, and Crohn's disease patient, I am fascinated by the connection between the brain and gut.

According to a *New York Times* article, the gut's brain, "known as the enteric nervous system, is located in sheaths of tissue lining the esophagus, stomach, small intestine and colon. Considered a single entity, it is a network of neurons, neurotransmitters and proteins that zap messages between neurons, support cells like those found in the brain proper and a complex circuitry that enables it to act independently, learn, remember and, as the saying goes, produce gut feelings."[1]

After reading the *New York Times* article, I came across Dr. Gershon's book, *The Second Brain*, when I was struggling with a diagnosis of irritable bowel syndrome. Dr. Gershon is chairman of the Department of Anatomy and Cell Biology at Columbia University's College of Physicians and Surgeons at the Columbia-Presbyterian Medical Center in New York City and is a pioneer in research related to the gut/brain relationship. In his book, he presents a fascinating combination of neuroscience and gastroenterology. Dr. Gershon has devoted thirty years of research to this "brain in our bowel" science, and his writing is persuasive and passionate.

Emeran Mayer, M.D. also theorizes that just as meditation calms the mind, it can also relax the bowel and promote healing. In his research clinic at UCLA, he has found that most patients notice an improvement almost immediately after starting to practice meditation.

In my meditation practice, I strive daily to "open up my heart," which is for some a symbolic act (or a spiritual affirmation) that reinforces my commitment to healing my self and reaching out to the world and the spiritual forces that I feel guide me. Since I am tall (almost 5 foot 9 inches), I sometimes slouch, and hold my shoulders inward; nowadays, I remember my dance training and pull my shoulders back, which helps me focus on opening my heart.

When I get those "butterflies" in my stomach—one example is having a client call you up and berate you over the phone if a publishing job is late (yes, this does happen, and once a client fired me after a weekend-long Crohn's flare-up!)—I sometimes tell my client to "please wait a moment," and I go sit on a pillow on the floor and take a few deep breaths and feel a weight lifted from my heart and abdomen; then, I pick up the phone.

I often use the following intention to end my yoga practice and also as an overall stress reducer: "May our thoughts be kind and clear; may our words and communication be kind and clear; may our actions and intentions be for the greater good of all human beings."

According to Phillip Moffitt in an article in *Yoga Journal* entitled "The Heart's Intention,"

"Setting intention, at least according to Buddhist teachings, is quite different than goal making. It is not oriented toward a future outcome. Instead, it is a path or practice that is focused on how you are 'being' in the present moment. Your attention is on the ever-present 'now' in the constantly changing flow of life."

CHAPTER 7

Influence of Lifestyle on IBD

PICTURE THIS . . . a woman and man gather greens from their garden. They come into the house, and she mixes together a simple oil and vinegar salad dressing while he washes the greens and starts to prepare a salad. To accompany her salad, she cooks some lightly steamed vegetables and whole grain rice. Their son is setting the table, and their daughter is washing dishes that accumulated while the meal was prepared. When the meal is ready, mother, father and the children gather at the table to have a nice dinner. They sit and eat and talk, taking their time to savor each bite. They are relaxed; there is no TV on and no computer in the background. They laugh over silly thoughts and share memories from their past. They are completely at peace as they enjoy time together, along with their vital, nourishing, and important meal.

Now ask yourself, how often do you think this happens for the average American? Rarely! In one study published in the *Archives of Family Medicine*, it was found that only half of all 9-year olds sat down with their families for dinner and only about a third of 14-year olds. For over ten years, the National Center on Addiction and Substance Abuse (CASA) at Columbia University has been conducting an annual study of family sit-down dinners and how they affect the health of children. They found that children who eat sit-down meals with their families are more likely to eat breakfast, consume more fruit, vegetables and dairy products, and tend to perform better in school. These children are also less likely to smoke or drink, experiment with drugs, become overweight, depressed or suicidal, or have erratic eating habits, eat fried food, or drink soda. A follow up study to this confirmed lessened drug experimentation in teenagers who ate regularly with their families.

Today, lack of proper time for meals, and, along with it, lack of time to properly chew and digest our food, has also become a significant trend within our society. This is directly affecting health, and, coupled with the poor quality of the food we consume, it is contributing to alarming weight gaining trends.

Simply put, the standard fast paced, TV watching, sedentary American diet and lifestyle that most people have become accustomed to is killing us, one by one. With the excess toxin load, excess stress, lack of movement, lack of proper time for meals, lack of emotional support, and lack of self-worth, we are generating life-killing habits.

It is time to start cherishing our bodies again. We must stop harboring the thought that we are "separate" from our bodies and cease encouraging this mentality by treating ourselves with suppressive drugs that only treat symptoms. Instead, we must focus on living healthfully. We should learn to listen to what our bodies are trying to tell us with the physical symptoms we experience and use that knowledge to live better. We must also be proactive in guarding our health so that we are less likely to become sick.

Every symptom that the body has is a key to understanding what is happening underneath; think of a symptom as a sign pointing towards a much bigger problem within us that, through the symptom, finally comes to the surface. Symptoms are truly the only way our body has to communicate with us and should be viewed as opportunities to look deeper within ourselves.

EXAMINING LIFESTYLE FOR TOTAL HEALTH

Treatment plans, whether or not they are naturopathic, must always focus on treatment of the whole person. This is true for those living with an illness or condition like IBD. If we do not address the whole person when facing an illness, the large obstacles to cure, left untreated, will continue to prevent an individual from attaining health and wellness.

Treating a whole person, whether healthy or living with an illness, means we must begin by taking a close look at how we live and be aware when our lifestyle is detrimental to us. For those with IBD, just like many other diseases, many lifestyle aspects are involved in the etiology of the condition. These include physical and emotional factors, among them: lack of movement or physical activity, lack of proper time for meals, lack of emotional support, lack of self-worth, and lack of body awareness.

PHYSICAL FACTORS INFLUENCING WELLNESS

Poor eating habits and a lack of an exercise routine go hand in hand to create major health problems for millions of Americans.

When it comes to health and the physical body, many of us may only think of accident or injury. Although many of us have had either minor or major physical stresses such as injuries and accidents, we must also be aware of how we treat our bodies on a daily basis. We often forget that the way we live every day also defines our physical health overall.

Lack of Physical Activity

Our society as a whole neglects exercise and experiences lack of overall physical activity. Rates of obesity have skyrocketed in recent years. According to statistics published by the Center for Disease Control (CDC) in 2008, only 1 state had obesity prevalence less than 20%. All other states had over 25% and six states had even greater than 30% for obesity prevalence.[1] This is huge. If a fourth to a third of our population is obese, then it is no wonder we have such rising rates of chronic illness! This information is proof that we are doing something wrong as a collective society and our lack of movement significantly contributes to our enormous obesity and chronic illness problem.

Dede's Experience

I am committed daily to getting exercise, and this is something I hardly did before my surgery. I have friends who are therapists who tease me and say I am "going overboard," but I just laugh at them. I also frequently tell my clients that I am going to be out running during my lunch break. When I go for a walk or run, I sometimes bring my iPod and listen to inspirational books on tape. Books like *Three Cups of Tea* by Greg Mortenson and David Oliver Relin; or *Mountains Beyond Mountains* by Tracy Kidder, are stories that give me hope and help me think "outside the box" of my own personal illness and suffering.

LACK OF EMOTIONAL SUPPORT

A lack of exercise contributes to poor health, and so does a lack of emotional support. When it comes to a discussion of disease, wellness, and the development of organ function and dysfunction as we age, the importance of affection and attention must never be understated.

It is said that "all we need is love." It turns out this is true: there is a great deal of research that supports that humans need love for survival and to maintain basic functions. In the book, *The General*

Theory of Love, authors and psychiatrists Thomas Lewis, Fari Amini, and Richard Lannon explain how we thrive based on physical contact and attention and how important social connection within our peer group is to living well. The authors offer an alternative view of neuroscience and the brain that is based on social behavior and love rather than the strictly neurological or chemical view.

This is why childhood development is so important when evaluating disease development in patients. During the initial complex developmental period of an infant's life, an infant wants and needs security, routine, touch, and love. These intimately social feelings are required by the infant for survival before the infant can even begin to understand their meanings. This means we are instinctively social beings, not by choice, but by being part of the human race. According to the National Child Abuse and Neglect Data System (NCANDS), an independent study by Prevent Child Abuse America estimated that over 1,750 children died of maltreatment in the United States in 2007 and at least 40% of these deaths were directly linked to neglect.

In Chapter 4, we took a closer look at childhood development and health. As we saw, lack of social and emotional support in early childhood development can lead to the development of future illnesses. And subsequently, lack of social and emotional support in adulthood can either lead to illnesses or exacerbate them: lack of affection and attention and love can lead to illness. For example, the famous Framingham Heart Study was performed in the 1950s to determine cardiovascular disease risk factors. This is when cholesterol was initially revealed as a significant risk to cardiovascular disease.[2] This same study found that another significant risk factor for cardiovascular disease is the lack of a significant other or partner. This proves that if we lose contact with other social beings, there is something that is not fulfilled within us that normally helps to maintain and keep vibrant our true life force, immune system, and all organ systems.

EMOTIONAL STRESS

Now let's move on to discuss a cause of inflammatory bowel disease around which there is some controversy and disagreement: emotional stress.

As many of us are aware, stress has a significant and impressionable influence on all diseases. In fact, stress and the hormones that are secreted in times of excess stress directly affect our aging. In today's world, our lifestyles play a huge role in the prevalence of particular diseases, including all chronic illnesses and cancer.

Stress is a controversial cause of IBD because there are conflicting studies on the relation of stress and IBD. However, when we look at the picture of IBD through pathophysiology and clinical experience, it is clear that stress is absolutely connected to IBD. Stress may not be the *cause* of IBD, but it is certain that many IBD sufferers who report their symptoms and condition reveal that their state worsens under stress. If you have IBD and are reading this text, you can most certainly attest to what is being suggested. Haven't you spent more time in the bathroom when you are under extreme stress? Physiologically, when a person is under stress, specific proteins such as pro-inflammatory cytokines, are released that promote inflammation within the body. In fact, according to an article published in *Neuro-immunomodulation*, chronic stress and aging have been shown to increase some of the same pro-inflammatory cytokines, especially IL-6 that are increased in IBD.[3]

Any chronic illness brings with it the complexities of the mind/body connection. Sometimes it is unknown whether the disturbance started in the mind and spiritual realm and then promoted dysfunction in the physical body or if the prolonged course of chronic illness, pain, and suffering created dysfunction in the mental, emotional, and spiritual realms. Women often experience disease differently. The willingness of a physician to accept the challenges and benefits that come with women having a surplus of uniquely feminine hormones is imperative to gaining wellness.

WOMEN AND CHRONIC DISEASE

Emeran A. Mayer, M.D., Professor, Departments of Medicine, Physiology, Psychiatry & Biobehavioral Sciences at the David Geffen School of Medicine, UCLA, directs the NIH-funded UCLA Center for Neurobiology of Stress. This unique Center aims to study the interactions of stress, pain, and emotion, and the role of sex related differences in these interactions, to better understand such common, complex disorders like irritable bowel syndrome and Interstitial cystitis. One integral focus of the Center (and why it relates so well with this book) is to study how complementary and alternative treatments such as the mind/body therapies are beneficial to aid in chronic disease. As a gastroenterologist, with a focus on neuroscience, Dr. Mayer is particularly interested in the research on women's relationship to chronic pain and disease and why they are more vulnerable as an area for study.

Dr. Mayer has a longstanding interest in clinical and neurobiology aspects of brain-gut interactions in health and disease. He has published more than 110 original articles, numerous review articles and chapters, co-edited two books and organized several interdisciplinary symposia in this area. Homeostasis and its disturbance in health and disease is of particular interest to Dr. Mayer's team, along with stress and its relationship to pain, as well as mind/body interactions as they relate to obesity, eating disorders, inflammatory and functional bowel disease, and psychiatric disorders. The inability to maintain homeostasis, which is the delicate balance of the body when faced with adverse conditions that can cause stress, is integral in bowel health in particular.

STRESS AND THE GUT

It is vital to address stress when mapping a path towards wellness for those living with IBD, Crohn's, and UC. Below, when we take a closer look at disease in our disease model, we specifically chart how the body reacts after stress: the brain increases ACTH, which in turn stimulates the adrenals to output cortisol and decrease DHEA, our anti-aging hormone. This increase in cortisol then decreases stomach acid and HCL and decreases pancreatic enzymes. These significant decreases, especially when occurring long term, have significant effects on GI health and overall body health. The decrease in HCL and pancreatic enzymes leads to undigested food in the small intestine, increases yeast and bacteria through the whole gastrointestinal lining, and can lead to mal-absorption and leaky gut. After this occurs, the liver has to increase its function to deal with the effects of poor digestion and unwanted fermentation.

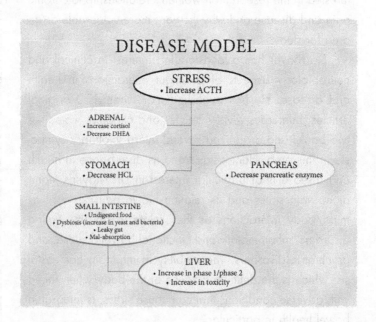

In addition, stress has detrimental effects on gastrointestinal health. Stress has been known to increase gastrointestinal lining permeability, which thus can increase allergy and inflammation potential. Stress also reduces visceral pain thresholds, which also can contribute to various psychosomatic disorders. Exposure to acute and chronic stressors has the ability to change ion exchange in the gut in addition to decreasing mucosal barrier defenses in the gut lining and promoting low level chronic inflammation. All of these previous alterations caused from acute and chronic stressors can lead to decreased pathogenic bacteria resistance, therefore allowing greater microbial multiplication.[4]

STRESS AND DEPRESSION

Stress is known to cause or contribute to various psychosomatic disorders such as anxiety and depression. According to a study published in the January 22, 2007 issue of the *Archives of Internal Medicine*, cynical thoughts, depressed moods, and chronic stress have a direct link to elevated inflammatory markers and increase risk for cardiovascular disease.[5] We can deduce that any emotions that increase inflammation are harmful to IBD patients and restrict or inhibit the ability of these patients to heal properly (more on depression as it affects IBD later on in this chapter).

PHYSICAL STRESS

When thinking of stress, most people generally categorize it as emotional. However, the word "stress" in relationship to the human body encompasses much more. Stress on our bodies can come from outside sources, as well.

As it affects the human body, stress can come in the form of environmental toxins such as plastics, pesticides, pollutants in the air, toxins in cigarettes, chemicals in drinking water and various other exogenous chemicals. Some of these we have direct control over and some of which we do not. Once harmful agents enter the body, the body's own metabolic wastes can further increase stress, especially in one's organs of detoxification if organs are not eliminating optimally or one's microbial balance is disrupted.

In summary, emotional problems such as stress related to one's occupation, family, deadlines, traffic, and any other emotional difficulty directly affect many body functions including immune response, brain function, and digestion. To add to that, physical stress also directly affects one's health.

MORE ABOUT STRESS AND IBD

Let's talk a little more on the physiology behind stress and how that can directly affect inflammatory bowel disease.

Within the nervous system, there are two different and contrasting systems: the *sympathetic system* and the *parasympathetic systems*. The parasympathetic system is responsible for digestion, rest, repair, and sexual function. The sympathetic system is responsible for our fight or flight response and also protects us during injuries/pain.

When a person is in pain, under chronic stress, or has a chronic illness, they are "sympathetic dominant," meaning the sympathetic system is the prominent system functioning at most times throughout the day. Continued sympathetic dominance severely inhibits a person's ability to heal due to lack of parasympathetic system functioning and leads to chronically elevated inflammation in the body. In summary, being aware of the effects of stress on the body is key for anyone with IBD.

EXPERIENCING DEPRESSION

Just as we must take a close look at stress as it relates to health, it is also extremely important when addressing IBD to also address depression, anxiety, or other psychosomatic disorders associated with disease.

With depression, sometimes it is hard to know when the disease is the cause of the depression or if the depression was the trigger to disease symptoms. No matter what the case may be, when dealing with IBD, a person may acquire symptoms associated with depression.

Depression often leads to or is a result of low serotonin levels. Low serotonin can increase the amount of pain an individual senses, can keep someone from being active, starting or maintaining treatment protocols, and most likely will interfere with sleep, which will affect healing. If depression is present and not addressed and only the GI tract is treated, then we may see an individual spiraling deeper into the illness because of the depression.

Dede's Experience

A gradual awakening and acceptance through psychotherapy is crucial to patients, especially those who have been newly diagnosed and feel fear, panic, depression, and loneliness—all common to sufferers of IBD. When I first started going to my therapist, Joseph M. Pumilia, Ed.D., I immediately felt safe in the room with him, overlooking a busy Main Street with the traffic sounds permeating the room in a dull background noise. I felt free to discuss issues like how a well-meaning friend urged me to go immediately on medication without really asking me about the serious discussions I had had with my husband and the countless hours of research and the anxiety associated with "going against a doctor's orders," especially in the case of such a respected doctor as Peter Banks, M.D.

I also discussed the embarrassment of not being able to travel. For example, on a long-planned vacation all the way to the Outer Banks with my family, I was stricken with a flare-up and spent the week in bed. Another time, I felt the embarrassment of having to change my underwear on an airplane and figure out what to do with the soiled pair. When flares occur and you have to beg your adolescent children to get you a cup of tea because your husband is sick of dealing with you, you can't help feeling exhausted and emotionally bereft. The list could go on and on, but suffice it to say, a therapist really helps! Not all my experiences were fraught with dire consequences, however, and we also have laughed in my support group about going to a party and immediately checking out where the bathrooms are in case of an emergency or having to explain over and over to people why I don't eat wheat, or corn, or mushrooms, etc.

To have a sympathetic ear and someone who is a licensed therapist with a Masters or Ph.D. is a great benefit. It is highly recommended for a spouse or partner, or parent of a child or teen with Crohn's or UC to also attend a private session with a therapist, if only occasionally, to check in about the stress of being a caregiver.

DYSFUNCTIONAL PATTERNS

For those living with IBD, negative thought patterns and behavior can cause major setbacks to healing. An important part of learning to live with a condition is recognizing negative patterns and stopping them—even when the illness itself leads individuals to detrimental ways of thinking.

Lack of Self-Worth and Caring for our Bodies

In our culture, many people live extremely fast paced lives. Patients often say that they don't have time for their illness or they don't have time to pay attention to what symptoms their body is presenting. Interestingly enough, symptoms are the way the body communicates, and if individuals don't listen, the symptoms get louder and more persistent until they force the individual to finally rest. Without body awareness, we see low self-esteem or self-worth, as well as many physical complaints including fatigue, headaches, and insomnia.

Dede's Experience

When I was in Costa Rica working as a chaperone for a college trip last year, our host told us that in Costa Rica, one rises with the sun and the animals in nature. Early in the morning at around 4:30 am, the birds make such a racket, and the cicadas are deafening. My first day there, I awoke in my single bed that was situated in an open-air bedroom that I shared with some of the other students. I had never heard such a racket. Especially the howler monkeys! After a day of physical work and hiking or horseback riding, as well as our work with students in the local *escuela*, we were exhausted and ready for bed. We had no electricity after dark, so our headlamps were used sparingly for reading only. The 3–4 books I brought with me were of no use while I was down there—I hardly read anything. I was too interested in the natural world, and the only books I read were natural histories or bird books.

That trip to Costa Rica helped teach me the importance of slowing down and becoming in tune with the pace of the natural world. This has been very beneficial while living with Crohn's because it helps to reduce one's stress levels, which can often wreak havoc on the intestines and GI tract.

Boundaries and the Gut

Another very important emotional connection to gut health is having proper boundaries. We view the gastrointestinal tract as the first line of defense against the materials of the outside world that are ingested by eating. It is the layer between our insides and what we are exposed to through what we ingest, such as food and drink. Its optimal function secures a healthy internal environment. Often times, physical aspects of our bodies follow emotional aspects.

When we can't digest our outside world, we often have a difficult time with digestion of our foods due to emotional distress. For example, this is often seen in children who have a new sibling enter the home; the addition of a brother or sister is often a very large adjustment for a child to take in (or "digest"), and sometimes stomach problems arise in the form of stomach aches, diarrhea, or other digestive complaints. It goes without saying that these children do not improve if *only* the gastrointestinal tract is addressed; in a case like this, the child who is struggling needs emotional support to put them back on track.

If one has improper ability to say no or has regularly skewed boundaries in relationships, this can be reflected in gastrointestinal boundaries and health. When considering treatment of inflammatory bowel disease, which is clearly an upset in the gastrointestinal boundary layer, it is of significant importance to address emotional boundaries. Working with patients on being able to say "No," if this is a problem, can help instill confidence and lead to faster healing of the gastrointestinal tract. Although there are no studies to support such a connection, it is seen very often clinically with gastrointestinal complaints.

PART II
Living with IBD

CHAPTER 8
Treatment Options

WHEN YOU or your loved one was first diagnosed with IBD, you probably felt like your life had taken a sudden spiral downward. You may have found yourself in a state of utter confusion, a deep-seated feeling of loneliness and depression taking root in the very core of your being. This may sound dramatic, but many sufferers of both Crohn's disease and ulcerative colitis feel this way in response to their diagnosis. The good news is that the better informed you become about your newly diagnosed condition or possible diagnosis, the better off you will be in the long run.

Dede's Experience

When one is newly diagnosed, one way to cope is to educate oneself as much as possible. I read everything I could get my hands on: Elaine Gottshak's book *Breaking the Vicious Cycle*, Dr. Rachel Naomi Remen's essays, *Kitchen Table Wisdom*, and Saki Santorelli's groundbreaking book, *Heal Thy Self: Lessons on Mindfulness in Medicine.*

LIVING WITH CROHN'S

The problem that many IBD sufferers know only too well is that these diseases, especially Crohn's disease, can reoccur. Although therapies can reduce signs and symptoms, often the hope for full remission is stymied by widely varying factors.

Dede's Experience

At the end of Part One, it was noted that there are many triggers that can cause IBD flares: for me they were diet, stress, smoking cigarettes (yes, I admit that I smoked for many years), and menstrual cycle.

Having been diagnosed with a moderate case of Crohn's disease that was classified by scarring of the terminal ileum (also known as fibrostenotic disease), I immediately went into a state of denial. I have since found that this type of reaction is common in patients when first diagnosed and, in fact, follows the stages of grief outlined in Elisabeth Kuhbler-Ross' book *On Death and Dying*, which presents 5 stages that terminally ill persons may go through upon learning of their terminal illness. The stages are: Denial, Anger, Bargaining, Depression, and Acceptance.[1]

So, denial came to me without any definitive form through reading. I went home to Vermont after my stay in Boston: home to my three children, my busy life running a business, and home to denial of living with a chronic, incurable disease like Crohn's disease.

Treatment options often include hospitalizations, surgery, and medications, but they rarely include a holistic approach that incorporates acupuncture, a new diet (potentially wheat-free), stress reduction, psychotherapy, yoga and meditation, naturopathic medicine, and a special protocol in detoxification.

Dede's Experience

I recently attended the Crohn's and Colitis Foundation of America and the Dartmouth-Hitchcock Inflammatory Bowel Disease Center's Symposium entitled, "Commonly Asked Questions about Crohn's and Colitis." The Symposium was completely sold out and there were people there with lots of questions about alternative and diet therapies to help them fight these diseases. The doctors all hoped that some of the alternative therapies (like the new refrigeration therapy, or the "eating worms" treatment) would work, but they all seemed skeptical. The only theory that piqued the interest of the pediatric gastroenterologist at the conference was the link between the spread of IBD in the developing world with the onset of refrigeration in the 1940s.

Treatment for any disease must first concentrate on increasing proper elimination through emunctory, or elimination, organs and facilitating optimal function of all internal glands and hormone systems. When the proper groundwork is set for healing, the treatments, lifestyle practices, and even pharmaceutical medications are much more effective at reducing symptoms and promoting healing of illnesses. Our bodies were meant to function as a whole, and treatment plans should always be directed at the whole body to achieve the desired effect: wellness.

Biologic agents are being developed and utilized with this premise in mind, as many of the drugs for IBD involve TNF-α inhibition, but newer drugs targeted at various other cytokines are currently in development. Additionally, still more agents are being investigated such as drugs that inhibit T helper activation, part of the immune system response that triggers the inflammatory cascade. The problem with these forms of treatments is that by suppression of our tumor fighter molecule, we have an increased risk for disease, illness, and cancer. Current statistics on cancer incidents reveal one in every three women and one in every two men will be plagued with cancer of some form during their lifetime.

One has to ask the question: Why do we want to suppress only one part of a very complex and dynamic process of immune system homeostasis? Why not work to balance the immune system by stimulating the proper cytokines and working towards an immune system homeostasis that is promoting wellness, rather than suppressing the overachiever molecules and leaving the host vulnerable to infections and even cancer?

DRAINING THE CUP

Let's go back to the overflowing cup analogy from Chapter 6. The very first thing to consider in designing and beginning a treatment plan is how full and overflowing the physical body, or cup in this analogy, is and how long it has been this way. Also consider what factors are affecting the body or filling the cup that can be controlled and changed. Remember, there are aspects in everyone's cup that we don't have the ability to alter, such as one's genetic inheritance and some environmental toxins, pollens, physical anomalies, etc.

Increasing proper elimination and supporting optimal internal organ function is the first part of healing and reducing total body load or "what is in the cup"; in essence, this facilitates drainage from the bottom of the cup by stimulating the function of important elimination organs. By increasing elimination, the body's capacity increases and can take things in without being so close to overflowing in symptoms.

REMOVING OBSTACLES TO A CURE

The three organs initially treated when addressing total body health including IBD are the liver, kidney, and gastrointestinal tract. The liver is responsible for breaking down many toxins within the body and is also responsible for making and breaking down all hormones in the body. The kidney helps to ensure proper filtration of all fluids in the body, excreting waste and maintaining proper blood pressure. The gastrointestinal tract is the first line of our immune defense against the outside world, helps us digest foods and absorb nutrients, stores serotonin (an important mood chemical in the body) and many white blood cells (important cells related to the immune response), and helps remove waste from the body.

By improving the function of all three of these organs, most people begin to feel better. Wastes are eliminated better, hormones are metabolized more regularly, and the foundation for health is begun. This, in addition to lifestyle and diet changes, needs to be in place before beginning specific Crohn's or digestive treatments in order for life changing and long lasting changes to occur.

Dede's Experience

During the months leading up to my surgery for a bowel obstruction, my health continued to worsen steadily. I developed gallstones and a very painful kidney stone, my energy was drained, and my legs cramped frequently (most likely due to the potassium deficiency). I also developed diabetes after I was put on steroids. It was a long, downhill journey, and there were times I wondered when my next health problem would arise. This is very common with IBD sufferers. Working with my naturopath and my acupuncturist to rebuild my organ function has taken time, and I still go to have "tune-ups" especially for my liver function, which is vital to maintaining good health.

Always do research to see if anything you might be doing or consuming is increasing the likelihood of disease progression. Most obstacles to cure that we have control over come in the form of diet and lifestyle choices or emotional or physical stress due to occupation, injury, loss of family member, etc.

MULTIFACTORIAL TREATMENT APPROACH
Integrative care

Integrative care combines the best in conventional or allopathic medicine and the best in natural or complementary medicine to provide a whole-body approach to healing. In many cases of inflammatory bowel disease, integrative care is superb. Patients may have an M.D. who manages any pharmaceutical medicines they are taking, but they may also have a naturopathic physician who manages their holistic treatment, ensuring proper organ function and natural treatment. Both physicians can work together to discuss proper blood tests, imaging, and exams that need to be performed in a regular fashion. In addition to physicians, patients may seek care from acupuncturists, chiropractic physicians, energy healers, and so on.

Other practitioners may benefit the patient with various adjunctive therapies. It is important that, when involving more than a couple practitioners, they either communicate or understand what the others are working on so they can work in unison with each other to promote healing and wellness in the patient.

The following sections will inform you of many allopathic and naturopathic treatment options. A discussion of current allopathic treatments will be introduced first.

ALLOPATHIC APPROACH TO INFLAMMATORY BOWEL DISEASE

Allopathic medicine refers to conventional medical care most often practiced by M.D. physicians. Health care providers work with IBD patients to determine the optimal combination of anti-inflammatory drugs to reduce symptoms, and to help avoid or post-pone surgery. Because the steroids commonly used to treat IBD can cause serious long-term side effects, alternative treatments are constantly being sought.

MEDICATIONS

In some cases, it may be necessary to utilize specialized medications to help relieve symptoms, reduce inflammation, and prevent exacerbations. Oftentimes, it is necessary to try several different treatments and/or combinations of medication to discover what works best for an individual. The following are a few of the medications most commonly used to treat IBD.

Aminosalicylates

These are antibiotic type drugs used in the initial treatment of many IBD sufferers. They help to kill off any overgrowth of abnormal bacteria and can help to reduce symptoms quickly, but must be followed by appropriate probiotics to prevent their need again. They help by minimizing bacterial growth in the small intestine caused by bowel narrowing (stricture), fistulas (which occur when there is an abnormal hole or passageway between two different types of epithelia tissue and can lead to improper passage of intestinal contents to areas where the content does not belong), and/or surgery. Researchers suggest that antibiotics may also help suppress the immune system, which can also be helpful, when used short term, in IBD and other gastrointestinal illnesses.

Immunosuppressants

Deliberately induced immunosuppression—to reduce activation of the immune system—is another first line of defense for IBD and other autoimmune diseases. Medications, such as azathioprine and 6-mercaptopurine, work to control symptoms.

Corticosteroids

Because they are fast acting, corticosteroids (for example, prednisone) are usually given for short periods of time to treat flare-ups. Their many potentially serious side effects make them unsuitable for long-term treatment. Side effects include, but are not limited to, weight gain, water retention, osteoporosis, diabetes, high blood pressure, increased susceptibility to infection due to immune suppression, cataracts, and psychosomatic disorders such as depression.

Immunomodulators

Immunomodulators are also prescribed in IBD treatment. They suppress the immune system but, unlike corticosteroids, they are slow to work. Immunomodulators have fewer side effects and can be taken over the long-term, or in combination with corticosteroids.

Biologic Therapies

TNF inhibitors, also known as biologics, are used to treat both Crohn's disease and ulcerative colitis. Biologics are proteins that block inflammation by affecting substances in the body such as pro-inflammatory cytokines. Remember that cytokines are molecules that regulate and control inflammation.

Remission is the goal of IBD treatment according to allopathic medicine. Once this remission state is achieved in a patient, then drugs can be reduced, changed, or eliminated as long as symptoms stay under control and close supervision by a physician occurs during the drug regimen change.

SURGERIES

Surgery should be a last resort treatment, but if the need arises, surgery may provide relief for some individuals. About 20% of ulcerative colitis sufferers will require surgery at some time in the course of their illness.[2] Approximately 75% of Crohn's disease patients who have disease in the small bowel will have surgery in the first 10 years after diagnosis. Unfortunately, if no other treatment is done, nearly 50% of those who have surgery will still have a reoccurrence of disease symptoms. The following is a list of possible surgical procedures that are used in IBD.

Some absolute indications for surgery in Crohn's disease are:

- Perforation with generalized peritonitis: Generalized peritonitis is inflammation of the peritoneum, the tissue that lines part of the abdominal cavity and other internal organs of the body such as the liver and intestines.
- Massive hemorrhage: Hemorrhage is when severe bleeding occurs, leading to risk of fatality.
- Carcinoma: Carcinoma is a form of cancerous growth of tissue.
- Fulminant or unresponsive acute severe colitis: Fulminant colitis is any colitis that has rapidly become progressively worse.

Some absolute indications for surgery in ulcerative colitis are:

- Toxic megacolon: Toxic megacolon occurs when a life-threatening widening of the colon occurs rapidly in any intestinal disease.

- Perforation: Perforation is a hole in the intestine that causes potentially life-threatening effects.
- Hemorrhage
- Severe colitis failing to respond to medical treatment

There are various complicated surgical options available these days, which continue to change and develop with the advancement of medical technique and technology. If you are experiencing significant symptoms or problems that either warrant immediate attention or have not responded to previous treatments, please consult your physician or a gastroenterologist about surgical options that may be right for you.

Dede's Experience

In May of 2006, I was hospitalized for three weeks for a dangerous bowel obstruction due to a flare up of Crohn's disease. They removed a large section of my Sigmoid colon along with an attached granuloma, terminal ileum, and secum. I began to experience the illness in April of that year, but had been diagnosed with the incurable disease, Crohn's, many years before.

I was admitted to Dartmouth-Hitchcock Medical Center on Monday, May 22, 2006 with a partial bowel obstruction. I was very sick when I was admitted. They almost put a nasal/gastric tube down my nose to try to help relieve the increasing pressure on my bowel, and the risk of perforation was high. As I lay on the gurney, listless and lethargic, my husband ushered in residents, doctors, surgical teams, nurses, and medical students. By this time, my bowel sounds must have become legendary in the Dartmouth-Hitchcock ER. My distended belly was swollen to that of a 5-month pregnant woman—the only simile I can think of was that it was the size of a basketball!

Just trying to lift my head off the pillow seemed like such an effort. I was too tired to care about brushing my teeth or reading the magazine on my bedside table. I had been in bed on and off for two full weeks. The pain in my belly had progressed from intermittent spasms to a dull roar. The obstruction was finally 'banding' across the top of my belly like a snake. My husband jokingly called it the 'alien' because it did indeed seem to have a life of its own. The noises were almost comic! The rumblings and gurgling of my belly (which is something many Crohn's sufferers know about) are often embarrassing. People say things like, "You must be hungry!"

This "rumble" or "growl" sometimes heard from the stomach is called borborygmus, and it is a normal part of digestion. It originates in the stomach or upper part of the small intestine as muscles contract to move food and digestive juices down the gastrointestinal tract. Rumbles may also occur when there is incomplete digestion of food that can lead to excess gas in the intestine. In humans this can be due to incomplete digestion of carbohydrate-containing foods including milk and other dairy products (lactose intolerance), gluten or protein in wheat, oats, barley, and rye (celiac disease), fruits, vegetables, beans, legumes, and high-fiber whole grains. In rare instances, excessive abdominal noise may be a sign of digestive disease, especially when accompanied by abdominal bloating, abdominal pain, diarrhea, or constipation.

One of my doctors on the GI team said that my lab tests were extremely good for someone as sick as I was. More importantly, he said I was "very well-informed" about Crohn's disease, and that I didn't have a lot of corollary symptoms such as mouth sores or infected eyes, which frequently flare up when the body's immune defenses are weakened. As he took my medical history, he was amazed to hear that I hadn't been on any medications since being diagnosed with my disease in 2001 nor had I ever taken any steroids to help with flare-ups in the past.

WHAT IS NATUROPATHIC MEDICINE?

As explained earlier, naturopathic doctors practice a system of therapy that relies on strict regimens of natural remedies to treat illness.

According to the Coalition for Natural Health, historically naturopaths "emphasized the use of hydrotherapy, nutrition, manipulation, herbs, or homeopathy, the goal for all practitioners of natural healing was to stimulate the body to heal itself. *Vis medicatrix naturae*, or the healing power of nature, remains central to naturopathic philosophy today."[3] Rather than trying to attack specific diseases, natural healers focus on cleansing and strengthening the body.

According to Renee Lang, N.D., one of the top naturopaths at the Cancer Center of America in Philadelphia, naturopathic medicine is defined primarily by its fundamental principles:

1. The Healing Power of Nature
2. Do No Harm
3. Identify and Treat the Cause
4. Treat the Whole Person
5. Physician as Teacher
6. Prevention is the Best Cure
7. Establish Health and Wellness

Methods and modalities are selected and applied based upon these principles in relationship to the individual needs of the patient. Naturopathic medical practice utilizes all methods of clinical and laboratory diagnostic testing including diagnostic radiology and other imaging techniques. Naturopathic physicians are primary care physicians and will refer patients to specialists when indicated.

Naturopathic medical treatment utilizes a variety of modalities including:

- Nutrition
- Botanical Medicine
- Homeopathy
- Counseling
- Lifestyle Management
- Naturopathic Physical Medicine
- Vitamin and Mineral Therapy

Naturopathic medicine involves distinct systems of primary health care—an art, science, philosophy, and medical practice of diagnosis, treatment, and prevention of illness involving the whole body. The diagnosis by a naturopathic physician may go much deeper than the primary diagnosis of inflammatory bowel disease. They may look into the causes of immune dysfunction, glandular weaknesses, organ insufficiencies, and so on to come up with a treatment plan that addresses all aspects of the patient's illness etiology.

In the development of personalized medicine, many contributing factors must be assessed including one's environment, one's development and childhood illnesses, microbial balance, psychosomatic disorders, physical demands, additional health complaints, genetics, vitality, willingness and commitment to healing, hormone balance, and so on.

A skilled practitioner will be able to assess all of the previously listed factors and determine how and when to intervene with treatments and lifestyle changes.

DEFINING AN N.D. AND THEIR TRAINING

A licensed Naturopathic physician (N.D.) attends a four-year graduate level naturopathic medical school. The education includes all of the same basic science courses as an M.D., along with holistic and nontoxic approaches to therapy with a strong emphasis on disease prevention and optimizing whole body wellness. In addition to a standard medical curriculum, the naturopathic physician is required to complete four years of training in clinical nutrition, homeopathic medicine, botanical medicine, naturopathic manipulation technique, and counseling. Naturopathic physicians take professional board exams in order to be licensed by a state or jurisdiction as a primary care, general practice physician.

Instead of merely suppressing symptoms, treatment of any condition must always be multifactoral for it to help improve wellness. Natural treatment options available now are extensive, and the amount of herbs, medicines, and supplements out there is overwhelming and confusing. Many times, having a directed plan by a naturopathic physician will help you gain wellness faster than trying to self-treat.

INSURANCE COVERAGE ISSUES

For many patients in the United States who are interested in starting a holistic approach to dealing with IBD or other auto-immune diseases, many states are providing good coverage of naturopathic physicians and other alternative medicine providers. However, it should be noted that there are states that do not yet license naturopaths. The U.S. Congress has created the National Center for Complementary and Alternative Medicine (NCCAM) as part of the National Institutes of Health. Check out their website at www.nccam.nih.gov for information on complementary and alternative medicine.

Dede's Experience

It can also be noted that my health insurance in Vermont covers my office visits and naturopathic care but not the supplements. Vermont has always been a progressive state, having had a supportive governor-physician, Dr. Howard Dean, for many years leading up to the bill licensing naturopaths in the state in 1992.

TYPES OF TREATMENTS USED BY NATUROPATHIC PHYSICIANS

The following are often used by naturopathic physicians to bring about wellness and facilitate healing: diet modification, herbal remedies, lifestyle changes including exercise, homeopathy including biotherapeutic drainage (UNDA numbers), plant stem cell therapy (also referred to as gemmotherapy), IV treatment, acupuncture, neural therapy, nutritional supplements including both oral and intravenous treatments if needed, energetic therapies, mental and emotional techniques and support. These treatments will be explored in depth in future chapters.

Dede's Experience

My naturopath has me on the following:

- Daily multi-vitamins
- Fish oil capsules (very good for inflammation and soothing the GI tract)
- Digestive enzymes (such as Butryn, or pancreatic enzymes)
- Vitamin C with Bioflavanoids (depending on my bowel tolerance)
- Probiotics (probiotic supplements can really help in the treatment of IBD)
- Flax seed to help with my constipation (I buy the flax seed at the natural foods co-op and keep the seeds in the fridge. Then, I use a coffee grinder and grind up a few spoonfuls to keep in the freezer to prevent the seeds from going bad. Once daily, I dissolve one large teaspoon of ground seeds in water and then drink another glass of water afterwards
- Homeopathic drops for calming stress
- Dietary aids like ginger, pineapple, and turmeric as anti-inflammatories. Miso and green tea are also great for maintaining electrolyte balance and strengthening my immune system

My naturopath also has me on a total "detox" regimen that includes castor oil packs, meditation (I use Rodney Yee's "AM Yoga" DVD, or try Jon Kabat-Zinn's wonderful collection of relaxation CDs), skin "sloughing" before shower (which entails roughing up your skin with a loofah sponge from your extremities toward your heart and encourages new cell growth), drinking plenty of water, regular exercise and daily yoga, counseling with a social worker or psychotherapist, weekly (free) REIKI and monthly massage visits, acupuncture sessions monthly, and physical therapy with integrative manual therapy-healing. A good attitude also helps. I regularly repeat to myself positive messages like, "Don't let this disease rule your life and get you down, but when you need to, 'Ask for Help!'"

The suggestions I receive from my naturopath are an attempt to enhance my body's natural elimination processes through the digestive system, kidneys, skin, liver, and lungs. All are essential to help me optimize elimination with minimal aggravation while also undergoing specific treatment suggestions with my gastroenterologist. I have found this support team and naturopathic/acupuncture treatment to be extremely effective as an aid that can dramatically lessen the physical effects of inflammatory bowel disease.

HOMEOPATHY

Born in Saxony in 1755, Dr. Samuel Hahnemann founded homoeopathy. Homeopathy has been used by many practitioners successfully since that time. Homeopathic remedies (also called homeopathics) are a system of medicine based on these three principles:

- Like cures like: "Like cures like" is based on a method of treating a disease with the materials derived from the toxic and injurious agent that caused the disease symptoms. We can use a small dose of that same agent on a very dilute level and stimulate the body to fight against the symptoms the agent creates if we are exposed to large doses of it. For example, the apis remedy is taken from the venom of a bee. We can use apis to help treat any medical problem that involves redness and swelling similar to the redness and swelling caused from bee stings.

- Minimal Dose: The remedy is taken in an extremely dilute form; normally one part of the remedy to around 1 trillion parts of water. In this dilute form, it can remind the body how to fight against certain diseases or problems.
- One Remedy Covers Many Symptoms: No matter how many symptoms are experienced usually only a few remedies or just one remedy is taken, and the remedy choice will be aimed at all the symptoms a patient is experiencing.

When using a remedy acutely, it is important to use it often, but never for a prolonged period of time daily. Generally, you should use a remedy for 3 days either 2–3 times per day during an acute symptom. If the remedy has not worked within 3 days, then it most likely is not going to help in this situation and another remedy should be chosen. When using a remedy long term for a chronic situation, then it should be used 3 times per week, preferably every other day. Remedies can be alternated with each other, but often a doctor won't prescribe more than two at a time. An example of how to effectively alternate two homeopathic remedies is every other day. One remedy can be taken on Mondays, Wednesdays, and Fridays, and the other remedy on Tuesdays, Thursdays, and Saturdays. On Sundays, you can choose one of the remedies or simply take that day off.

Homeopathic remedies can be purchased in a health food store, obtained from many alternative practitioners, or can be found in the health food section of most larger grocery stores. If some homeopathic remedies can't be found in stores, they can be ordered online. A good site is abchomeopathy.com.

Examples of homeopathic remedies that can be helpful in digestive complaints include the following:

- Aloe is a great diarrhea remedy, especially when the diarrhea is sudden, explosive, and with a lot of flatulence that occurs while having the bowel movement.
- Alumina is a good remedy for constipation that is unresponsive to many other treatments.
- Apis is a great remedy to be used in chronic inflammation. It is great for swollen abdomen, inflammation in the colon, inflammation or ulcers in the mouth, and many other inflammations.
- Arsenicum is helpful in diarrhea, especially diarrhea that occurs from anxiety type reactions. Arsenicum can be used acutely with good response in acute diarrhea. Chronic worry that leads to chronic diarrhea responds well to arsenicum.
- Belladonna can be used in acute illness that occurs quickly. Usually the problems that come when a patient needs belladonna, come very quickly and need to be treated aggressively. Belladonna can be used in acute diarrhea or acute fevers.
- Carbo veg is helpful in many cases of flatulence. It is extremely helpful in colic, gas cases in infants, and for overindulgence of foods causing flatulence. In cases of chronic flatulence, carbo veg can be used long term every other day until the flatulence resolves.
- Calcarea carbonica is also a good remedy for individuals having various digestive issues that stem from sluggish digestion and sluggish metabolism. It is often used as a long-term remedy rather than acutely.
- Ignatia is a great remedy for grief and stress. Any past grief history that causes worry and stress can affect the digestive function and inflammatory bowel symptoms. Ignatia can be used acutely for a recent grief such as death in the family or loss of a loved one or can be used for chronic grief as well.
- Lycopodium is helpful when flatulence is significant. Most patients who can be helped with lycopodium also have a good appetite or often feel hungry, but are easily satiated when eating.

Lycopodium is a great remedy when ailments occur that are related to liver issues or biliousness.

- Nux vomica is a remedy that is helpful when constipation or ailments occur following ingestion of disagreeable foods. It is also helpful if reflux or heartburn is present. Most likely nux vomica also helps to treat aggression and aggravated states with anger or insomnia.

- Phosphorus can be used in rectal bleeding. It can be used acutely but also can be used in chronic rectal bleeds or intestinal bleeds even when the bleeding is not visible. As a general remedy, it can help soothe colitis.

- Podophyllum is also helpful in diarrhea.

- Sepia can be useful in cases of fissures, fistulas, and hemorrhoids. Sepia is also useful in rectal itching.

UNDA Numbers and Biotherapeutic Drainage

Biotherapeutic drainage uses homeopathy and plant preparations such as UNDA numbers to enhance the body's normal routes of elimination and improve cellular function. UNDA numbers were created in France over 50 years ago by Georges Discri. The name UNDA was derived from undulating water waves that carry medicine. UNDA numbers are made with homeopathic preparations of plants and minerals and are used to specifically target specialized tissues and stimulate their function. By opening routes of elimination and improving organ function, impurities are excreted, minimizing stress on the system and promoting better internal health. By improving proper elimination, the body is able to tolerate more external stressors without creating uncomfortable symptoms. UNDA numbers are the perfect remedies to begin cleansing with because they facilitate detoxification at a pace that the body chooses rather than doing harsh cleansing programs on a body that isn't prepared or doesn't have enough vitality to withstand the detoxification process.

By stimulating the body's elimination organs to function prop-erly, the body gets to choose what needs support. For example, by stimulating the enzyme systems within the liver, then the body's liver essentially chooses what processes it needs to improve within the liver to facilitate better health. So an 87 year old woman might utilize a liver UNDA number to help with elimination, a 2 month old infant may use the same liver UNDA number to help with hor-mone manufacture, and a 32 year old woman might use the same UNDA number to help with uniquely female hormone balance and cholesterol production. That is what makes these therapies truly unique. They themselves are individualized therapies; they are very "per-person" medications due to their selective varying actions in different individuals. The same liver remedy can be used with 20 different people and get different effects based on what problems they have. Also, these remedies are used monthly and build upon prior prescriptions. Therefore, one month, the liver, kidney, and gastrointestinal tract will be stimulated and supported while the next month, building upon the work that has already been accom-plished, the remedies chosen might stimulate deeper into those same organs or other systems may be supported depending on the patient's need.

UNDA numbers can be directed towards specific tissues or organs within the body promoting adequate function even if the function of that tissue or organ has already been compromised, degenerated, or damaged.

Most often, response to UNDAs is quick and revitalizing. In rare cases, initially the UNDA numbers and/or homeopathic remedies used for drainage may produce aggravation or symptoms of old disease conditions as the tissues are cleansed of previously incomplete healing. Usually the symptoms are not serious and even those who are sensitive can tolerate this process. These cleansing symptoms should be tolerated if possible, and they will usually last only 3–5 days.

During the cleansing and reprogramming process, the patient must focus on adequate nutrition, rest, exercise, water, sunshine, detoxification, prayer, positive attitude and expectation, forgiveness, and appreciation. Such ongoing activities and attitudes are the foundations of health and are discussed in Chapter 10.

These remedies are non-toxic, will not interfere with other medications (conventional or non-conventional), have a gentle yet deep acting and long lasting effect, and are safe for all ages including infants.

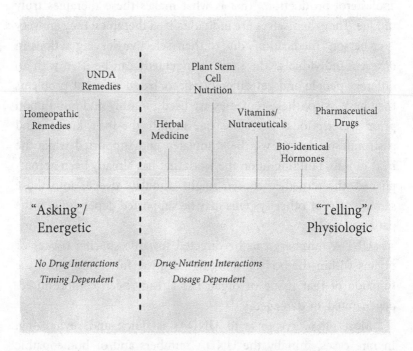

Remedies vary from "asking" the body to respond, to "telling" the body to respond. "Asking" remedies never interfere with other medications. Remedies that affect physiology have the potential for drug/nutrient interactions and drug overdoses.

This chart can be used to describe the effect UNDAs produce in the body. This chart symbolizes a continuum of "asking" to "telling" remedies or "energetic" to "physiological" remedies. An example of a strong physiologic remedy is any pharmaceutical drug such as effexor. 75 mg of effexor is 75 mg. The body has no ability to not respond to this 75 mg of drug. Therefore, more dosage causes more effect (and more side effects, for that matter). The higher the dosage, the more physiology is stimulated causing more effect. That is why we have such problems with drug overdoses and drug-drug interactions. The further on the continuum towards the left, the less directly physiologic the therapies listed on this chart are. For example, herbal medicine has the potential to cause physiologic reactions but is not nearly as strong physiologically as pharmaceutical medications. Beyond the dotted line towards the right, the medicines listed pose potential drug-nutrient or nutrient-nutrient interactions due to their physiological effects. UNDA numbers and homeopathic remedies, because they are only reminders to the body on how to function, don't pose any risk for nutrient-nutrient or nutrient-drug interactions. Because of this, they are safe to use with any medications and are safe with any supplements. There are no contraindications to the use of UNDA therapies except a strong alcohol allergy or strong alcohol addiction, which may be triggered by the use of small amounts of alcohol.

But because of their low physiological response, they are asking the body to perform a function rather than telling it. Therefore, they do work best when they are taken three times daily. It is not how much of the UNDAs that are taken, it is the continual reminder three times per day that make them effective at reminding the body how to carry out its functions.

TREATMENT OF PSYCHOSOMATIC DISORDERS

SAMe

SAMe can be helpful in the treatment of depression. It acts as a methyl donor and can help the body to complete and maximize its nerve connections in the brain. SAMe has antioxidant activity therefore will help to reduce free radical damage within the body. SAMe can help the body's methyl metabolism improve, therefore functioning to increase energy, improve cognitive function, and decrease pain. SAMe has also been used to treat osteoarthritis; response tends to be noticed within the first month of use. Insomnia, anxiety, or mania states can be associated with overuse of SAMe. Begin with moderate dosages and decrease if any of these are experienced.

Do not use SAMe with other antidepressant medications, especially selective serotonin reuptake inhibitors (or SSRIs). It may cause life-threatening symptoms (including agitation, tremors, anxiety, rapid heartbeats, difficulty breathing, diarrhea, shivering, muscle stiffness, and excessive sweating). Insomnia is also an unwanted side effect of combining these drugs.

SAMe dosage: 400 mg daily

5 HTP

Another great over the counter treatment for depression is 5 HTP. 5 HTP is a serotonin precursor and can help the body to make more serotonin and leave the available serotonin in synapses for a longer period of time, therefore directly affecting mood and warding off depressive symptoms. 5 HTP can also help with insomnia, agitation, fatigue, and lack of motivation. It is often helpful in chronic pain situations because it increases sleep needed for healing, improves mood, and decreases sensation of pain.

Again, 5 HTP should not be used with other antidepressant medications, especially selective serotonin reuptake inhibitors, or SSRIs. Serious side effects can result. Results are seen as quickly as with SAMe but are definitely noticeable.

5 HTP dosage: 100 mg two times daily

Magnesium

Magnesium is an all-time favorite nutritional supplement. From stress to muscle cramps to premenstrual cramps to migraines, to constipation, magnesium can benefit most people. The only deter-ring factor in the use of magnesium for inflammatory bowel disease is during diarrhea states. Magnesium can induce diarrhea states in most individuals after a certain dosage. Usually this is around 800 mg. Patients should take the highest dosage that they can take with-out getting diarrhea. In most people this comfortable dosage lies around 600–750 mg per day in two divided dosages. Magnesium can help regulate proper bowel function, reduce stress, prevent and treat anxiety, improve sleep and prevent migraines. Magnesium can be used daily and long-term. There is no toxicity to magnesium, therefore rare risks are involved with the use of magnesium.

Magnesium is contraindicated in those with renal failure and those who have myasthenia gravis. It is also contraindicated in those with high-grade atrioventricular (AV) blocks unless those with high-grade AV blocks have artificial pacemakers.

Magnesium dosage: 600–750 mg daily in two doses

L-theanine

L-theanine is a particular amino acid that is helpful in the treat-ment of anxiety and often improves sleep. Amino acids are building blocks of proteins and specifically L-theanine simulates the body's production of alpha brain waves, creating a state of deep relaxation and mental alertness. This same alertness coupled with relaxation is what is often experienced after meditation. L-theanine can also increase GABA, an inhibitory neurotransmitter responsible for in-hibiting excess excitation and therefore inducing relaxed states and sleep. L-theanine is quicker acting, therefore should be taken at least two times, but possible three times in significant anxiety.

L-theanine dosage: 50–100 mg two times daily

Psychosomatic drugs may be indicated if needed to treat severe anxiety or depression. Seek out the advice of a qualified physician if you feel you are suffering from depression and anxiety that is not responding. Untreated significant depression can impede healing results to other therapies directed at the gastrointestinal tract.

PHYSICAL MEDICINE CARE

Cranial sacral is a subtle type of body work that can help to reset much of the nerve input to the gastrointestinal tract. The cranio-sacral system comprises the membranes which surround the central nervous system (the brain and spinal cord), the bones of the cranium and sacrum, the tissue that surrounds all of the nerves and nerve pathways in the body, and the cercbro-spinal fluid, a lubricating fluid produced within the central nervous system for protection. Every organ, muscle, and tissue is linked to this system and cranial sacral body works to correct any imbalances so that proper nerve input to organs can improve. Specific work on the gastrointestinal tract can improve nerve communication in and out of the gastrointestinal tract in order to facilitate better communication with the central nervous system. Many massage therapists may do this procedure or could refer you to someone who does.

Chiropractic care becomes important in some patients. Chiropractic care can relieve congestion in the spine, help to re-align vertebrae, and can help to promote more optimal gastrointestinal function due to its corrective abilities in the spine, which is where all of the nerve roots exist for carrying information to and from the GI tract.

Massage can be extremely beneficial due to its ability to move lymphatic fluids, increase circulation, promote healing, and provide stress relief and relaxation. Most often, illness is exacerbated by stressful lifestyles and massage is able to force patients to slow down even if for an hour, and relax with no outside stimulation.

Dede's Experience

I try to have a massage once a month because it fully rejuvenates my body, even on a cellular/skin level. Kim Timlege, my massage therapist, offers discounts when you buy a package of massages, so I take advantage of sales. She does a deep tissue and trigger-point massage therapy that is proving to be beneficial and curative. I feel rejuvenated and the benefits of massage are immediate, including peace of mind. Caregivers can learn some basic massage techniques and purchase massage oils to try at home as well.

Neural therapy is one of the most effective physical modalities due to its profound and lasting results. Neural therapy, a form of mesotherapy, is a treatment that is used to treat chronic pain and chronic illness. This therapy was first developed in Germany and is currently most prominently used throughout many European countries. There are physicians within the United States using this therapy. Neural therapy uses non-toxic medications, is quick acting, has limited side effects, reverses the disease process, restores tissue to its normal functioning state, and offers long lasting results.

The neural therapy procedure is easily administered because it is a non-invasive procedure, which consists of micro-injections of medications into and under the skin, allowing small amounts of medicine to be delivered to the site of injury without affecting the rest of the body. The non-toxic medications consist of the local anesthetic procaine and specific plant derived homeopathic medications. Neural therapy is unique in that the specific applications of the medicines into the skin or dermis where there is a high concentration of nerves, allowing for a time-release dosing system, which allows for both immediate and long-term relief of symptoms. This application can provide relief from weeks to months and even years when the injections are performed correctly. While this procedure is effective for any person suffering from pain, athletes and people who are active especially appreciate this procedure because of neural therapy's quick acting results with limited side effects and no systemic damage that is too commonly seen with oral pain relief medications.

Neural therapy shifts the body into a more parasympathetic state promoting healing and repair. Injections into nerve areas that reflex to internal organs help to facilitate a proper resting state and optimal nerve function, re-setting the proper peripheral communication so that the body can again see itself, as well.

Neural therapy injections help to drain inflammation by flushing lymphatic tissue, stimulating white blood cells to promote healing, and providing nutrition to soft tissue for healing.

One of the very special and unique qualities of neural therapy, specifically with the use of procaine, is that procaine is metabolized into DMAE and PABA, which are nutritive to the nerves, act as co-factors to help facilitate metabolism, offer anti-oxidant support, and have anti-aging qualities. Most importantly, these nutrients can be directed to specific areas by an experienced physician; this is a technique that is extremely exclusive and individualized to the patient that cannot be attained by taking these nutrients orally. In colitis, there are specific colon injection areas that can be injected in addition to injecting the kidney and liver areas for increasing elimination.

ACUPUNCTURE AND ACUPRESSURE

Acupuncture is a method of encouraging the body to promote natural healing and to improve functioning. Inserting needles and applying heat or electrical stimulation at very precise acupuncture points is the basis for this type of treatment. The classical Chinese explanation for this is that channels of energy run in regular patterns through the body and over its surface. These energy channels, called meridians, are like rivers flowing through the body to irrigate and nourish the tissues. An obstruction in the movement of these energy rivers is like a dam that backs up the flow of water.

According to the American Academy of Medical Acupuncture's website (medical acupuncture.org), the meridians can be influenced by inserting needles in the acupuncture points so that the acupuncture needles unblock the obstructions at the dams, and reestablish the regular flow through the meridians. Acupuncture treatments can therefore help the body's internal organs to correct imbalances in digestion, absorption, and energy production activities, and in the circulation of energy through the meridians.

The modern scientific explanation is that needling the acupuncture points stimulates the nervous system to release chemicals in the muscles, spinal cord, and brain. These chemicals will either change the experience of pain, or they will trigger the release of other chemicals and hormones which influence the body's own internal regulating system.

The improved energy and biochemical balance produced by acupuncture results in stimulating the body's natural healing abilities, and in promoting physical and emotional well-being.

Try to go monthly to a local acupuncturist—this really helps!
Continue the acupuncture and naturopathic treatment even
if you inevitably have to go on maintenance drug therapy
as well.

FINDING A QUALIFIED PRACTITIONER

*(from The National Center for Complementary and
Alternative Medicine)*
Health care providers can be a resource for referral to acupuncturists, and some conventional medical practitioners—
including physicians and dentists—practice acupuncture.
In addition, national acupuncture organizations (which can
be found through libraries or Web search engines) may
provide referrals to acupuncturists.

- CHECK A PRACTITIONER'S CREDENTIALS. Most states require a
  license to practice acupuncture; however, education
  and training standards and requirements for obtaining
  a license to practice vary from state to state. Although a
  license does not ensure quality of care, it does indicate
  that the practitioner meets certain standards regarding
  the knowledge and use of acupuncture.

- DO NOT RELY ON A DIAGNOSIS OF DISEASE BY AN ACUPUNCTURE
  PRACTITIONER WHO DOES NOT HAVE SUBSTANTIAL CONVENTIONAL
  MEDICAL TRAINING. If you have received a diagnosis from
  a doctor, you may wish to ask your doctor whether
  acupuncture might help.

A NOTE FROM DEDE'S ACUPUNCTURIST, JANET SINCLAIR

According to Dede's acupuncturist, Janet Sinclair, "What is interesting about acupuncture is the philosophy, or even art, that informs the medicine. The simple and deepest idea is yin-yang theory, which is an observation that the active parts of our lives and the quiet parts of our lives need to be in balance to promote health and well being. The active and quiet aspects exist in every cell of our bodies, every organ system, and between various organ systems. Patterns of harmony and disharmony have been observed over thousands of years, and when an acupuncturist is trying to understand how to best treat their patient, he or she is looking at these patterns."

In the case of any digestive illness, it is likely that the stomach and spleen energies are not in a correct relationship to each other. It most likely is also the case that another organ system is then thrown out of balance as well, often related to the liver energy, which deals with stress. These imbalances co-arise. In the case of the stomach and spleen energies, on a physical level this means that the body may not be comfortable enough to properly receive and absorb nutrients, and otherwise may not be able to metabolize those nutrients to build tissue and create energy. On an emotional level, these energies are related to the balance of one's reception to receiving and enjoying the experiences that one encounters, and then whether or not the person is likely to return the generosities that he or she has received. In everyday life, this would equate to a person's ability to both give and take.

When acupuncture is used to treat the patient, each aspect of a particular yin-yang balance is addressed. This means that the person is assisted at the level of individual cells, the specific organ systems involved in the disharmony, and a possible distortion in a person's existential stance and corresponding belief system that he or she operates from.

Dede's Experience:

My Monthly Acupuncture Routine

When I go to my monthly acupuncture session with my practitioner, we talk about my health during the past month, and she makes notes. It is important to feel relaxed and safe in any new medical or alternative therapeutic environment, and with my practitioner, I feel like I am getting free mental health therapy. She is so thorough and compassionate in her holistic treatment of someone living with an incurable digestive disease. After the health update, I lie on the table and immediately start to relax and unwind while she gently takes my pulse and asks me questions about how I am feeling. It is amazing how much she can tell by taking my pulse! She then inserts tiny, relatively painless, needles into a few key points around my body, usually in the extremities.

Sometimes it is uncomfortable, but the pain only lasts for a second and the anticipation of the needle going in is worse than the actual pain itself! I often laughed at my inability to deal with the "pre-pain" of the treatments, and whenever I was uncomfortable, my practitioner would always switch to using an herb called "moxa" instead of a needle (moxa is the common herb mugwort—this is like a roadside weed—and it is heated which stimulates circulation around the area and in turn stimulates *chi,* or energy, to be used for overall health and healing). As I learned, the pain only lasts for a few seconds after the needle goes in and then it disappears gradually. She always encourages me to speak up if something is too painful, as that really would not be beneficial.

I find the relaxation I feel while lying there on the table is something I look forward to each month. I often fall asleep on the table!

Below are a few valuable points that are extremely helpful in balancing meridian energies that flow through particular organ systems. All-important to digestion and gastrointestinal health, the following points can be massaged daily with a deep massaging into the specific point: LV 3, GB 41, LI 4.

Sometimes a directional massage is helpful such as for LV 3 and GB 41 points. It is beneficial to move the energy through these points to the outside. To do this, begin by massaging at these points and moving outward towards the toe crease as if to move the energy away, releasing stored tension and energy. Begin between the bones that lead up to each toe and move deeply through the tissue, feeling the stretch and stimulation.

GB 41 is located between the fourth and fifth metatarsal bones—in the indentation between the bones leading up to the toes. GB 41 is mostly indicated in headache and some abdominal pain disorders[4] and can facilitate better and more efficient gall bladder function.

LV 3 is located between the fourth and fifth metatarsal bones—in the indentation between the bones leading up to the toes. LV 3 is a liver point and can provide balancing for all liver pathologies. LV 3 can be helpful in menstrual problems, digestive problems, and can also be helpful in headaches. It is a calming point therefore can be helpful for anxiety, anger, and insomnia. When it is used with LI 4, also called the four gates treatment, it powerfully affects the flow of blood and energy in the body.

LI 4 is located on the back of the hand, between the 1st and 2nd metacarpal bones (first and second fingers) right in the web of the fingers. It is useful in people who have gastric pain, abdominal pain, constipation, diarrhea, and dysentery. It is also useful in many complaints related to the head such as headache, dizziness, congestion, swelling and pain of the eye, sinusitis, epistaxis (nosebleed), toothache in the lower jaw, and swelling of the face. When it is used with LV 3 (the four gates), because it affects the movement of the Qi and blood in the body, it is helpful in eliminating stagnation and alleviating pain.

Daily massage and stimulation of these points will increase blood flow, help improve the effectiveness of your current therapies, improve mood, decrease inflammation, and promote healing.

AT-HOME ACUPUNCTURE

Here are seven painless and simple at-home acupuncture steps you can do to maintain good health and vitality.

1. BRUSH YOUR GUMS AND TONGUE. Spend at least 5 minutes each time you brush (longer is even better). Set a timer because 5 minutes may seem like a very long time at first. The acupuncture points along the gums match with the entire body system, as does the tongue.

2. BRUSH YOUR SCALP. Remember when moms insisted that we always brush our hair for 50 strokes? Turns out, there are hundreds of acupuncture points on the scalp itself. For a quick session, massage the governing vessel 20. This point is located at the very top of the head, the point of 100 meet-

ing points, which enables you to access several channels at once. Spend time massaging your scalp with your fingernails and even while you shampoo.

3. PUSH BACK YOUR CUTICLES ON YOUR FINGERS AND TOES. Just the act of pushing back your cuticles stimulates acupuncture points that go *directly* to every muscle and tendon in the body, bringing on relaxation. Need to keep a small child quiet at an event? This works like a charm. Plus you can trace every finger front and back as well.

4. LOOFAH YOUR BODY. This is a hard sponge that softens with use. Loofah plants can be grown, and are much softer than those found at most department stores. (Note: when purchasing a loofah, be sure it says 'loofah' on the package.) Use the loofah wherever there is skin. There are thousands of acupuncture points all over the body. If you find a sore or itchy spot, spend extra time there. It is likely that it is an acupuncture point that needs stimulation. Electricity is accumulating there and stimulation via massaging or using a loofah disperses this accumulation. Before showering, use the loofah sponge to aggressively rub from the extremities toward the head, beginning with the arms, then working up from the feet. After you rub all the dead cells off your body, an invigorating shower further energizes you and allows for the stimulation of new cell growth.

5. MOISTEN YOUR NASAL MEMBRANES. When you splash water on your face, keep water on your little fingers. Put your little fingers inside your nose and moisten all around. You do not need to sniff water up into your sinuses. Moistening your nasal membranes increases your chi (your body's bio-electrical energy).

e

6. BREATHING EXERCISES. Most of us are chest breathers, rather than abdominal breathers, so we tend to breathe shallow most of the day. On inspiration (breathing in), push your stomach out as far as you can. On expiration (breathing out), let your stomach fall back to neutral. This is very difficult to do at first without thinking about it. When you breathe with your abdomen it forces the diaphragm to drop and thus increases your lung capacity. This is why singers practice breathing so that they are able to sustain notes much longer. Breathing leads to more oxygen, more chi and more energy.

7. MASSAGE YOUR FACE, HANDS, FEET, AND EARS. You can do this yourself, but it is more relaxing and fun if done by someone else. These areas also treat the entire body individually.

(List by Patricia S. Wesley, D.C., of Wesley Chiropractic)

These seven relaxation techniques are really easy to do at home. Foot massages are also very beneficial, as well as candle-lit hot baths with lavender oil drops in the water.

HERBAL REMEDIES

Herbal medicine has been used for centuries to treat various conditions. In fact, many drugs are derived from plant based medicines or herbal constituents. Herbal medicines for inflammatory bowel disease combine anti-inflammatory herbs, demulcents, astringents, immune enhancing herbs, and adaptogens.

Anti-inflammatory Herbs

Turmeric, or *curcumin*, can be used as a spice in foods or can be taken in therapeutic doses either through tincture form or capsule form. Curcumin has significant anti-inflammatory properties and very high antioxidant capability making it a superb nutrient to use in any gastrointestinal condition, inflammation related condition, and to use preventatively to ward off cancer and chronic illness.

One of the most effective forms of curcumin is to take it in a tincture with ginger. Dr. Black's clinic uses a tincture called the "anti-inflammatory tincture," which is used for anything from inflammatory bowel disease to arthritis to acute injuries to chronic idiopathic inflammatory diseases. This tincture gets extremely positive results in almost all patients who begin taking it regularly. The proportion should be about 50/50 curcumin to ginger as they are both anti-inflammatory and the ginger helps with the absorption of curcumin. Because curcumin is poorly absorbed, it should be complexed either with ginger or bromelain for optimal absorption and optimal effects.

In people who have ulcerative colitis, previous studies have shown that curcumin supplements, when compared with placebo, reduced the number of relapses by about fifty percent. A recent article in *Current Pharmaceutical Design* also notes that in the treatment of inflammatory bowel disease, curcumin "and its unrivalled safety profile suggest that it has bright prospects."[5]

Turmeric complexed with ginger in liquid tincture form: 2 dropperfuls 3–4 times per day. Too much curcumin can cause stomach upset so don't use much more than this listed dosage. In capsule form, curcumin complexed with either ginger or bromelain can be taken at 500 mg of the curcumin 2–3 times daily. If you can't find a capsule of curcumin and ginger or curcumin and bromelain, you can always buy curcumin and ginger capsules separately and take them together to help with curcumas absorption and reduce gastrointestinal irritation.

Ginger can also be used alone especially for gastrointestinal irritation and inflammation. Ginger tea is helpful in settling the stomach and can also be helpful in nausea. The tea should be used at 3 cups daily.

Garlic is also a useful supplement especially if there is concern that there is yeast, bacterial, or parasitic overgrowth. Garlic is anti-inflammatory, blood thinning, antimicrobial, and anti-cancer. Garlic supplements need to be taken with the odor to get the best effect. Don't bother buying an odor-less garlic supplement, because you lose half of what makes garlic so powerful. If your stomach, family members, and co-workers can handle it, the best way to take garlic is to eat garlic cloves. One way to do this is by making a small drink.

Garlic Drink Recipe

> 1 clove garlic, minced small
> ½ glass filtered water
> pure maple syrup
> juice of half a lemon

Mix together and drink 1 of these drinks two times daily.

Try just eating garlic, as it is becoming more studied for its health effects and its reduction in colorectal cancer risk in inflammatory bowel disease sufferers. Though, if you want to take garlic in capsule form, the proper dosage should be at least 900 mg daily. Some supplements can be found having high allicin content, which is the main constituent in garlic. These high allicin supplements are different than taking garlic supplements therefore the mg dosage daily is much smaller.

Yucca is a plant native to Mexico and Southwestern United States. Yucca has been known in folk medicine as a treatment of arthritis and inflammatory ailments. Native American Tribes and native peoples of Mexico have proclaimed many uses of Yucca that have dated back hundreds of years. Yucca is comprised of many phytochemicals that make it special for use in many conditions. Some of the important phytochemicals are phenolic compounds such as resveratrol. Resveratrol is an important anti-inflammatory agent that helps reduce aging and helps to keep inflammation under control. The phenolic compounds in yucca also act as anti-oxidants or free radical scavengers which act to reduce damage and inflammation caused by free radicals, thereby reducing damage and aging of tissues, joints, organs, etc . . . [6] Yucca is more often used in patients who have inflammatory bowel issues or gastrointestinal distress that coincides with arthritis. Yucca is also high in saponins, which play a part in complexing with the cholesterol molecule in the body aiding in cholesterol lowering. This cholesterol lowering effect was demonstrated more than 45 years ago.[7,8]

Yucca dosage should be two 500 mg tablets or capsule 2–3 times per day. It is always best to start at a lower dosage and increase if no result is seen. Yucca can also be found as a tea and will be mentioned in the tea section as well. The usual dosage for tea is 3–5 cups per day. Long term high dosage use of yucca extract can result in interference with the absorption of vitamins A, D, E, and K.

Pau d'arco, or *Tebebuia impetiginosa,* contains at least 20 active compounds, including naphthaquinones, anthraquinones, alkaloids, quercetin, and other flavonoids. Flavonoids will help support and balance the immune response and inflammatory response and help to reduce the allergic response. Alkaloids are found in varying quantities in most plants and are the part of the plant that makes them have a bitter taste. Because large dosages of alkaloids can be toxic, this bitter taste, obviously more bitter in more toxic plants, can warn animals of the plant's toxic nature. This is one example why it is most helpful to use plants in their whole form as much as possible for treating illness. Using plants in their whole form will help ensure the amounts of toxic or irritating substances like alkaloids can be in a dosage appropriate surrounded by other balancing phytochemicals for producing subtle and effective medicinal effects. Alkaloids are a nitrogen containing part of the plant that represent a very diverse group of significant compounds that include well-known drugs like the opiates, caffeine, nicotine, and quinine, the anti-malarial drug.

Pau d'arco can be used as an immune system stimulant, and to decrease inflammation. It should only be used in inflammatory bowel disease patients if there is an underlying infection problem contributing to illness.

Pau d'arco can be found in capsules, tinctures, or as a tea. The tea is best, but it must be boiled slowly to gain all medicinal properties from the plant. The following dosages for capsules and tinctures should be discussed with your doctor prior to use:

- Capsules: 300–500 mg three times per day
- Tincture (1:5)*: 0.5–1 mL (about ⅛–¼ teaspoon) two or three times per day

To prepare pau d'arco tea, mix 3–6 tablespoons of the inner bark tea with one quart of cold distilled water into a teapot. This can be brought to a low boil for 20 minutes. Then strain and drink 3 cups daily.

Even low doses of pau d'arco can cause dizziness, nausea, vomiting, and diarrhea and can interfere with blood clotting. It may also cause skin sensitivity. The potential for drug-nutrient or nutrient-nutrient interactions should be considered when using pau d'arco. Don't use with other blood thinners unless supervised by a physician and if any side effects occur after its use, discontinue. Pau d'arco should be avoided in pregnancy and lactation. Pau d'arco should not be given to infants or children.

Cat's claw is a large woody vine indigenous to the Amazon rain forest of South America and is also known as *Uncaria tomentosa*. Its phytochemical makeup is important to its functions as well. The active compounds in cat's claw include alkaloids, triterpenes, phytosterols, and proanthocyanidins. Some of the phytochemicals in cat's claw appear to have anti-inflammatory, antioxidant and anticancer

---

* The 1/5 pertains to 1 part of dry herb to 5 parts alcohol for extracting the medicinal properties of the plant.

effects.[9] It is used in a wide variety of health issues including healing and treating digestive and intestinal disorders. The phytosterol component of the herb provides insight into how it can balance the immune response. Phytosterols are components of plants that are responsible in balancing the actions of the Th1 and Th2 systems, mentioned in earlier chapters and can play a significant role in reducing inflammation by balancing any over-active or under-active part of the immune response.

Bitters

Bitters are useful herbs that function to stimulate gastric function in addition to liver function and detoxification, they help to control blood sugar, and they aid in stress relief due to their stimulation of the parasympathic nerves in the gastrointestinal tract. They are helpful in IBD patients because they stimulate mucosal immunity and function to create balance of inflammation within the GI tract and they may help to repair mucosal wall damage caused by inflammation.

Examples of bitters include licorice, peppermint, calendula, dandelion, artichoke leaf, blessed thistle, angelica, motherwort, wormwood, bitter orange peel, lemon peel, gentian root, mugwort, goldenseal, cascara sagrada, hops, chamomile, and yarrow.

An example of how to use bitters is before or after a meal. It can be in the form of a tincture or tea, but tincture is best considering it is easier to carry with you when you are out. A tincture of equal parts licorice, dandelion, and blessed thistle might be a good start. Use 2 dropperfuls with each meal. This may have to be taken in a little bit of water due to its strong and bitter taste.

Demulcents

A demulcent is an herb that functions in providing a soothing film over a mucus membrane. For example, honey is often used as a demulcent for a sore throat, because it helps to coat the throat mucus membrane. Respiratory demulcent herbs can be extremely effective in treating coughs and soothing lung irritation.

As mentioned earlier in the enema and suppository section, the demulcent slippery elm can be very useful in calming, soothing, and coating the GI tract. Other soothing demulcents include comfrey, althaea, licorice, and matricaria, which can be used to help soothe gastrointestinal irritation.

Demulcents can be used as cold teas, tinctures, and capsules. It is best to use demulcents as warm or cold teas because they perform best that way.

Astringents

An astringent is used to help bring tissue together. It shrinks it together and can help with micro tears, micro bleeds, and excess mucus in the gastrointestinal tract. Some helpful astringents in IBD include agrimony, comfrey, geranium, yarrow, and lady's mantle. Most often, these are not used alone, but are used in combination with anti-inflammatory herbs, demulcents, and immune enhancing herbs.

Immune Enhancing Herbs

One of the most important areas to support in autoimmune diseases is the immune system. We sometimes wrongly direct our treatments for autoimmune diseases by suppressing the immune response rather than balancing the immune response. Drugs targeted at T-lymphocyte regulation will be a fairly large area of research in the future. For now, we utilize herbs that help the body achieve better immune homeostasis such as astragulus, baical skullcap, chaparral, pau d'arco, albizia, reishi, shiitake, and other mushrooms.

One must be careful and skilled at using herbal medicine to treat the immune system in autoimmune diseases to ensure proper stimulation without over-stimulating the wrong part of the immune system.

Adaptogens

Adaptogens refers to a class of herbs that help the body in its adaptation to its environment. Most of the time, adaptogens help to support the adrenal gland, which sits on top of the kidney and functions in our stress response. The adrenal glands help to control immune function, blood pressure, emotions, blood sugar, and importantly, control the output of our cortisol, which helps us feel energy for the day and modulates our immune response. Adaptogens are very useful in the beginning of illness to bring energy up, help individuals cope with stress, and to improve sense of wellbeing and sense of worth. This increased self-awareness and self love helps patients focus on their treatment plans and increases compliance with new lifestyle and diet changes.

Examples of adaptogens are Siberian ginseng, withania, licorice, astragulus, rehmania, codonopsis, maca, rhodiola, schisandra, cordyceps, reishi mushroom, and Noni. Use adaptogens in tincture form. Pick 2–4 herbs to add to a tincture in equal parts and dosing it at 2 dropperfuls 3 times per day. The last dose of the day should not be before bed, as adaptogens can often keep individuals from sleeping well.

Example adaptogen tincture for IBD:
> 1 part Siberian ginseng
> 1 part maca
> 1 part rehmania
> 1 part codonopsis due to its affect on the gastrointestinal tract

If you can't find an herbalist or doctor who can make this tincture, then you can purchase four 1-ounce tinctures and mix them together into a 4-ounce dark container. Then you can pour 1 ounce back into one of the bottles, label it appropriately and this can be your dispensing bottle. If you can't find one of these herbs, then replace it with another of the adaptogens listed or omit it entirely. Before making an adaptogen formula read about the specifics of each adaptogen and determine which 3–4 adaptogens are most appropriate for you.

TEAS FOR HEALING
IBD Tea for Mood, Nervine and Calming

> 1 part St. John's wort (St. John's wort should not be used by people currently taking anti-depressant medication)
> 1 part lemon balm
> 1 part passionflower

Steep 1 tablespoon per 10 ounces of water. Bring appropriate amount of water to boil, remove from heat, add dry herb, cover, and allow to steep for 15 minutes. Strain through fine tea strainer, cheesecloth, or clean nylon/T-shirt. Drink 3 cups daily. You can make up to 90 ounces at once and sweeten with honey if desired. If you are making bigger batches it is perfectly okay to store in the refrigerator and drink chilled.

IBD Tea for Detoxification and Soothing

> 1 part licorice root
> 1 part marshmallow root
> 1 part burdock root
> 1 part dandelion root
> 1 part yellow dock root

*Yellow dock should not be used by people taking drugs that decrease blood calcium, such as diuretics, Dilantin, Miacalcin, or Mithracin. It also should not be used by people with kidney disease, liver disease, or an electrolyte abnormality.

Because these herbs are roots, the tea needs to be boiled to release the maximum medicinal qualities of the herbs. Add 1 table-spoon of the root mixture to 10 ounces of water. Bring water with herbs to a boil and boil for 10 minutes, remove from heat, cover, and allow to sit for 15 minutes. Strain and drink 3 cups daily. You can make up to 90 ounces at once and sweeten with honey if desired. If you are making bigger batches it is perfectly okay to store in the refrigerator and drink chilled.

IBD Tea for Inflammation and Immunity

1 part pau d'arco
1 part cat's claw
1 part ginger root–grated fine
1 part chaparral

Steep 1 tablespoon of the mixture per 14 ounces of water. Bring appropriate amount of water to boil, remove from heat, add dry herb, cover, and allow to steep for 15 minutes. Strain through fine tea strainer, cheesecloth, or clean nylon/T-shirt. Drink 3 cups daily. You can make up to 90 ounces at once and sweeten with honey if desired. If you are making bigger batches it is perfectly okay to store in the refrigerator and drink chilled.

IBD Soothing GI Tea

Peppermint (Should not be used in people with heartburn or reflux)
Chamomile

Steep 1 tablespoon per 10 ounces of water. Bring appropriate amount of water to boil, remove from heat, add dry herb, cover, and allow to steep for 15 minutes. Strain through fine tea strainer, cheesecloth, or clean nylon/T-shirt. Drink 3 cups daily. You can make up to 90 ounces at once and sweeten with honey if desired. If you are making bigger batches it is perfectly okay to store in the refrigerator and drink chilled.

IBD Gas Relief Tea

> 1 part fennel seeds–grind in coffee grinder slightly to help break apart the seed
> 1 part fenugreek seeds–grind in coffee grinder slightly to help break apart the seed
> 1 part althaea (marshmallow) root
> 1 part slippery elm bark–grind or break apart

Because these herbs are roots, seeds, and barks, the tea needs to be boiled to release the maximum medicinal qualities of the herbs. Add 1 tablespoon of the mixture to 10 ounces of water. Bring water with herbs to a boil and boil for 5–10 minutes, remove from heat, cover, and allow to sit for 15 minutes. Strain and drink 3 cups daily. You can make up to 90 ounces at once and sweeten with honey if desired. If you are making bigger batches it is perfectly okay to store in the refrigerator and drink chilled.

NUTRITIONAL POWDERS

Beneficial nutritional powders include spirulina, kelp, protein powders, brewer's yeast, ground nuts and seeds, acai powder, green tea powder, greens powder, ground milk thistle seeds, and ground nettle powder. The following is a short list of average dosages of each nutritional powder. As with everything, more is not always better. Moderation is the key to health; therefore do not begin including each of these powders in addition to many or all of the supplements listed.

Spirulina is a variety of seaweed that contains trace elements and minerals, essential fatty acids, increases absorption of iron and stimulates the immune system, cleanses and detoxifies, gently removes heavy metals, has enzymatic activity, is a vegetarian source of B-12 and contains a significant amount of beta carotene.

1 rounded tablespoon 2–3 times per day, this comes to around 30 g daily. It is often suggested that you can take up to 100 grams daily. You can add this to water or smoothie or juice and it doesn't change the taste significantly, but certainly affects the color. My favorite way to consume spirulina is by drinking what we term in our home, "green lemonade."

Green Lemonade Recipe

    1 cup filtered water
    1 heaping tablespoon spirulina powder
    ½ teaspoon juice from a lemon
    ½ teaspoon pure maple syrup or agave syrup
    Stevia can be substituted for the sweetener in this case easily

Blend all together in the blender until mixed. Enjoy 3 times per day (you can multiply the recipe by 3 to make 1 days worth). Make fresh every day.

Kelp is another variety of seaweed and the powder can be beneficial to the gastrointestinal system due to its potential to regulate the thyroid, which is the organ that sets the pace of enzyme function in the body. The thyroid is our battery. How well it is functioning determines how optimally our enzymes can function. Remember that enzymes are important in the gastrointestinal tract for digesting foods and absorbing nutrients in addition to facilitating many metabolic reactions occurring within the gastrointestinal system, immune system, and the rest of the body. There are many health claims regarding the regular use of kelp including alleviating arthritis pain, increasing energy levels, stimulating immunity, improving glandular function, appetite control and weight loss most likely due to optimizing metabolism. Kelp has been used to treat thyroid deficiency due to its rich iodine content. Kelp can help with poor digestion, flatulence, constipation, and helps to support mucus membrane health, which might give proof to its positive effect in inflammatory bowel disease patients. Kelp does have a distinct taste that is slightly salty. It can be used over food once daily.

Kelp powder: ½ teaspoon–1 teaspoon daily

Do not use if you have hyperthyroidism. Individuals who have hypothyroidism or borderline hypothyroidism may benefit most from daily use of kelp powder. The use of kelp may interfere with thyroid medication dosage requirements, therefore addition of daily kelp should be discussed with your physician and repeat thyroid tests should be performed six weeks after initiating kelp treatment.

Protein powders make a great addition for patients who need extra nutrition or need help balancing blood sugar. A protein shake can be added as a midmorning snack in between breakfast and lunch and can help to maintain stable blood sugars, stable moods, increased energy, and increased calories nutrition for nutrient-deficient patients.

Brewer's yeast can be used to sprinkle over popcorn and most savory dishes. Brewer's yeast is made from *Saccharomyces cerevisiae*. Brewer's yeast is high in B vitamins, chromium, and many minerals. Due to its high chromium content, it may be helpful in reducing and balancing blood glucose levels and has also shown benefits in improving poor lipid profiles such as high cholesterol. Adults can use 1–2 tablespoons daily, but you might prefer to use brewer's yeast for a nutritive additive to some of your foods, rather than something that is consumed every day. There are much better supplements specific to lowering glucose or cholesterol.

Ground nuts and seeds can be added to many foods. You can use ground nuts and seeds for anything from raw dessert crusts, to pancakes, to crispy snack balls, to toppings for savory dishes. They add quality protein and fat to many recipes and are easily accessible at your local grocery store. Make sure to buy fresh nuts and seeds and organic if possible. Many nuts and seeds are also high in mineral content and will offer good sources of calcium and magnesium and many other important minerals.

Ground milk thistle seeds and ground nettle powder can be fun and beneficial additives to your foods. These powders can be mixed with salt to make a healthy seasoning for the table. Milk thistle helps to support liver function and nettle helps to support kidney function.

Good for your Soul Salt:

> 1 part ground milk thistle seeds
> 1 part ground nettle powder
> 1 part sea salt

Mix together and store in salt shaker. Enjoy generously over food. This seasoning can be changed to fit your needs. For example, you can add kelp powder, sesame seeds, acai powder, and others to suit your needs and tastes.

BERRIES

Berries, with their exquisite healing properties, have flooded the health product market in recent years. From goji berries to acai to the proanthocyanidins found in blueberries, the healing properties of high anti-oxidant berries are on the forefront of antioxidant supplements. When researching berries and their health benefits, we learn the way they provide such good benefits is by scavenging up free radicals in the body. When left undisturbed in the body, these free radicals would normally cause tissue damage and destruction, aging, cancer, and other chronic illnesses. While some of these are normal processes such as aging, taking antioxidants can help to ward off the aging process and protect from chronic illness. Antioxidants also play a key role in the healing process and can be extremely helpful in digestive disorders due to its support of the gastrointestinal lining health. How strong an antioxidant is can now be rated on a scale according to its ORAC (oxygen radical absorbance capacity) content. The higher the ORAC content, the more potent of an antioxidant it is.

Using berries in a powdered form either in capsule or powder is my preference in addition to including them generously in the diet if available. For example, acai berries do not transport well from areas of Brazil to this country, therefore they are picked and immediately either pureed and frozen or they are freeze dried into a powder. Acai powder is a high antioxidant and nutritious powder providing a good source of healthy fats, fibers and proteins. Acai powder tends to rate very high on the ORAC scale but can vary depending on the manufacturer.

A safe goal for dosing berries, berry supplements, and berry powders is to look for ORAC content. Use an ORAC content of at least 3000 units per day.

Green tea powder is useful in patients for its antioxidant content. It does have caffeine and can also help with fatigue in the initial part of treatment if patients are feeling unmotivated and feel no initiation. It is also helpful for increasing cognitive function and inducing a sharper functioning mind. It can be mixed with frozen acai packets into a morning smoothie. Green tea has been shown to modulate the immune response and can help to control unnecessary inflammation.[10] There are numerous studies using green tea that reveal anticancer activity.[11, 12]

Smoothie Recipe

1 teaspoon green tea powder
1 packet acai pulp, unsweetened
1 cup filtered water
1 cup filtered 100% juice
2 tablespoons ground flax seeds

Blend until liquid. Drink chilled.

BENEFITS OF GREEN TEA POWDER

Regular green tea powder supplements can also provide added nutrition and antioxidant support for individuals with poor diets or poor digestion. Green tea powders can be added to smoothies or simply taken in water and can provide up to 10 servings of fruits and vegetables. They are not intended, though to take the place of eating fruits and vegetables. Anyone can use them daily, especially weak individuals who need the additional nutrition support. Most of Dr. Black's patients use them, but usually not in a daily form. Green tea powders can be added creatively to many foods, sweet treats, and juices. They will change the color and sometimes the taste depending on what type you purchase.

SUPPLEMENTS

Probiotic supplementation in Crohn's patients was seen to influence the mucosa immune system and actually change gene expression to increase a cytokine that is responsible for helping guide a natural and healthy oral tolerance. They claim this is the first evidence of its kind relating probiotics to genetic expression![13]

Acidophilus: supplementation proves beneficial in irritable bowel sufferers at decreasing diarrhea and reestablishing proper flora balance.[14]

A different probiotic, *Faecalibacterium prausnitzii* was studied in France for the treatment of Crohn's disease and proved beneficial in reducing inflammation in the colon.[15]

Fish oil is one of the best ways to increase essential fatty acids for reducing inflammation. Fish oils not only are beneficial because they help to balance inflammation in the gut, but they help to support all pathways within the body that depend on essential fatty acid metabolism. Clinically seen, the more healthy fat we consume, the increasingly healthy our body's fat balance becomes. Therefore, it is even easier to maintain a healthy weight if consuming essential fatty acids on a daily basis.

Dosing fish oils can be complex. Some fish oils are higher in EPA and some are higher in DHA. To get the most anti-inflammatory content in fish oil, it is important for the EPA amount to be high. The higher the EPA content and the colder of the water the fish lived, the higher quality of fat it had to make. This EPA content provides us with great inflammation protection. In general, we can consume fish oil as a supportive treatment or a therapeutic treatment. Fish oils other than cod liver oil can be used in high doses with patients initially to decrease their inflammation rather quickly.

For example, an initial starting dosage of fish oil in a colitis patient is often 2250 mg of omega 3 fatty acids (1050 mg EPA to 750 mg DHA) three times daily. Once the patient's inflammation calms down, this dosage can be decreased to 2250 mg of omega 3 fatty acids daily.

Digestive enzymes can be helpful for many individuals because they can remove stress from the gastrointestinal tract. During stress and inflammation, people have suppressed enzyme capacity in their gut, therefore supplementing with enzymes can promote better digestion and better breakdown of food metabolites. This better digestion leads to better absorption and less risk of increased vascular permeability due to unwanted stomach irritants such as larger food particles as a result of poor digestion.

Sachharomyces boulardi is a very important probiotic to use in times of excess yeast or chronic fungal infections. Many specialized tests can be used to check for unwanted fungi and yeast species in the gut. If an overgrowth of pathogenic fungi or yeasts are found, using saccharomyces can help by settling into the areas within the gastrointestinal tract that are normally inhabited by yeast and fungus species. Same with the use of bacterial probiotic crowding out pathogenic bacteria, probiotic yeast can move into and compete for survival within the GI tract with pathogenic or overpopulated yeasts and fungi. If yeast infections or fungi overgrowth are strong, only supplementing with saccharomyces may not be effective. If you try this supplement and do not notice improvement, then you may need a stronger medication to help kill the yeast or fungi species before adding back in the probiotic. Consult a physician if you need more support in this area.

DHEA: The use of DHEA over the counter is very poorly understood. Many to most DHEA supplements found in stores offer dosages of 25 mg or more. When using DHEA, many times the optimal and maximum dose is around 10–20 mg. DHEA is best when a protocol of slow increases can be observed over a period of weeks. This allows people to determine their best dosage. Start with 5 mg daily for 1 week and increase by 5 mg weekly. The dosages can be split between 2 times per day; a morning dosage around 9 am and an afternoon dosage around 1 pm.

DHEA is a hormone and though hormones should be avoided unless needed, sometimes hormones can be extremely beneficial. DHEA can be particularly effective in reducing inflammation, preventing chronic diseases and supporting adrenal and hormone production/function.[16] If you do not understand the use of DHEA and don't know that you have a deficiency, avoid the use of DHEA. If you have overt adrenal deficiency and low DHEA, and have tried many other treatments without success, DHEA could benefit you.

As with all hormones it is important to take them at the same time each day. When beginning the DHEA protocol, begin with 5 mg in the morning for 1 week. The following week increase to 10 mg, but take 5 mg in the morning and 5 mg in the afternoon time. On the third week, increase by another 5 mg by adding it to the morning dosage and the fourth week add the extra 5 mg to the afternoon dosage. So on and so forth until you find the week that you feel best. The maximum dosage is often 20 mg for individuals so if there is no change or you continue to feel well as you increase, then 20 mg is a safe place to stop.

WEEK	DHEA AM DOSAGE	DHEA PM DOSAGE
	9 am	1 pm
1	5 mg	0
2	5 mg	5 mg
3	10 mg	5 mg
4	10 mg	10 mg
5	15 mg	10 mg

Oftentimes, when they first start this ramping up DHEA protocol, individuals will continue to improve weekly, and as they increase the dosage will come to a week that they don't feel as well. This is how the dosage can be found. This is the week that was too much dosage. For example, if someone is taking it weekly and is feeling good and improved each week but feels more tired and not quite right during week 4, then 20 mg was too much DHEA for them.

This individual's daily dosage should now be 15 mg. Make a chart of how you feel each week including factors such as energy, bowel function, sleep, and overall sense of wellbeing. By keeping this chart and referring to it, you will be able to pinpoint the best dosage for you. Most likely it will fall between 10 and 20 mg daily. Be consistent with the time at which you take it daily.

Vitamins: A complex multivitamin and other vitamins such as vitamin D, vitamin K, and vitamin A can be helpful after the colon has been healed and bowel function is normal. Hold off on particular vitamins until the gastrointestinal tract is functioning better and has a better ability to utilize and break down the vitamins.

Minerals are also very helpful and can help to support nervous system function among many other things. Mineral absorption in compromised gastrointestinal function may not be optimal, therefore it is best to use single minerals at first if needed and reserve multi-mineral supplements to be implemented later as a maintenance plan. Single minerals may be more beneficial during initial treatment based on need and deficiency.

One of the minerals that is an exception to this rule is magnesium. Magnesium will often cause diarrhea in most people at around 800 mg daily; therefore patients should take the highest dosage that they are able to tolerate daily without getting diarrhea. For most people, this dosage turns out to be around 600–750 mg daily, divided into 2 doses. For migraine sufferers, the dosage can often be more, close to 1200 mg daily, without causing diarrhea and significantly helping with migraine symptoms.

Amino acids, which are the building blocks of proteins, can be beneficial in the treatment of inflammatory bowel disease. One helpful gastrointestinal amino acid is L-glutamine as it has a significant effect on colitis and other gastrointestinal symptoms. L-glutamine is known for its supply of nitrogen and help in restoring muscle mass in individuals who work out. Aside from this rebuilding of muscle, L-glutamine helps to repair the important and intricate functioning of the barrier lining of the gastrointestinal tract. It helps to keep the gap junctions tight, reducing the amount of larger particles entering the blood stream due to regular or consistent excessive mucosa inflammation. Gap junctions refer to the intimate encounter between two cells lining the gastrointestinal tract. This secure junction is what forms the virtually impenetrable passageway to the blood stream. L-glutamine also helps to increase the number of friendly or helpful probiotic bacteria within the GI lining.[17] Because of its stimulation of growth hormone, L-glutamine may also be helpful in aging effects. L-glutamine can be used up to 4 grams daily.

Other basic supplements may be needed in the treatment of IBD due to poor nutrient absorption. Here is a list of a few supplements and dosages. Oftentimes, it is more important to support with herbal formulas to decrease inflammation and improve gastrointestinal function prior to supplementing. In addition, if the IBD is controlled, then most likely a very good multivitamin can be enough complexed with consistent herbal and supplemental support.

- Folic acid: 800 mcg daily
- B complex and/or B 12:
- Beta carotene: 20,000 IU daily
- Vitamin D: 2000–4000 IU daily
- Buffered Vitamin C: 2 grams daily
- Vitamin E: 800 IU daily

IV NUTRIENT THERAPY

Sometimes individuals have such compromised digestion that they lack proper nutrients. If patients are severely malnourished due to their colitis, IV therapy can be very beneficial for energy, supporting organ function, improving metabolism, and decreasing inflammation. IV therapy should be given by a qualified practitioner. Many naturopathic physicians use IV therapy in addition to some medical doctors. The IV treatments should be focused on providing valuable nutrients or antioxidants and not on chelation, which is administering agents into the blood stream that force elimination of heavy metals in addition to important minerals, or other depleting IVs. Most of these IVs are drip procedures in which you would need to be in the clinic for 2-3 hours receiving your vitamin nutrition right into your blood stream. This is important for individuals with lack of proper digestion and absorption capabilities. Some IV therapy treatments can be shorter push-type IVs that take only minutes and can still restore some helpful needed nutrients.

If IV therapy is not available, then B-12 or B complex injections may provide the extra support you need if you are malnourished. Most physicians can do these or give you a prescription for them so that you are taught how to give yourself B injections at home.

IV therapy should not be the only therapy we rely on for healing. Though it can provide immediate relief and improved sense of wellbeing in patients, the underlying environment must be treated and balanced to prevent dependency on IV treatments for maintaining wellness.

TEAM OF SUPPORT

In many cases, more serious or aggressive care becomes extremely important. Depending on the severity of inflammatory bowel disease, some patients may need steroid support, surgery, and other interventions while they are working on a wellness plan. Healing does not happen over night and sometimes, it takes a very long time for treatments to help. We relate it to turning a very large ship around and going back upstream. It is very easy for the boat to drift downstream, but extremely more difficult to go against the current. It is a continual and daily effort for wellness, but extremely gratifying and well worth the effort when wellness is achieved.

Again, in order for all healers and practitioners working with a patient to work together well, it is important for all involved to have regular communication. This communication can be as simple as sharing blood test results, chart notes, treatment plans, etc. so the patient is well cared for and nothing slips through the cracks. Never think you cannot tell your medical doctor that you want to try naturopathic medicine.

An effective support team may include:

- Naturopathic doctor
- GI (it's important to find one who listens to you and knows about your life)
- Yoga teacher (obviously all "alternative team members" should be professionally trained and accredited)
- Acupuncturist
- REIKI and massage therapist
- Counselor or psychotherapist (to help with stress and psychological problems from your past and/or associated with work and current family stress from your disease)

It is important to interview the members of your support team and find out how they work and make sure you feel compatible with them. You can research GI doctors and hospitals on their websites to make sure they are current members of national organizations such as the Crohn's & Colitis Foundation, so you can be sure they are up-to-date on research. New patients can also go directly to the CCFA website and search for a doctor there.

The National Institutes of Health also sees the need for complementary or alternative treatments in IBD. Posted in June of 2008, Rush University Medical Center began two research studies evaluating dietary changes and complementary medicine for the treatment of IBD, funded by the National Institutes of Health. One study is determining the impact of mind/body medicine on ulcerative colitis patients and the other study is looking at the impact of how diet can affect Crohn's disease patients.[18] Dr. Ali Keshavarzian, director of digestive diseases and nutrition at Rush and principal investigator and co-investigator on the studies, reports that over 40% of IBD patients are already using some form of alternative care.

MONETARY CONCERNS IN USING ALTERNATIVE THERAPY

Many patients diagnosed with IBD question how they will manage to pay for alternative treatment—a logical question, especially because some insurance companies do not cover these types of treatments. There are many resources available through the CCFA and local hospital support groups—not just for money, but also for programs like "community supported acupuncture" on a sliding-fee scale. Also, scheduling monthly visits with your practitioner can lower the fee slightly, because some practitioners and clinicians appreciate the steady work and will discount their rate.

Supplements can also become fairly expensive, but they do last a long time and many naturopaths will work with their patients to calculate the minimum effective doses that can be used while also saving your pocketbook—other therapies, like massage, are also costly and can average $50–70 per visit; however, these, too, can be budgeted and reduced.

You can also buy a massage book and some oil and learn to give massages to your spouse or partner, thereby saving money! However, going to a licensed massage therapist is really worthwhile, especially when one is newly diagnosed or in need of direct support to help with pain management or stress. As a way to maintain health, massage can be considered a luxury. It is also an ancient form of healing that dates back to the Ayurveda traditional Indian system of medicine. Massage therapies are frequently turning up in intensive care units and pain clinics, as well as birthing rooms in hospitals.

Hospital stays and surgeries are typically very expensive even with health insurance, but these can be paid off over time through a payment plan with the hospital.

Some insurance companies are very encouraging and supportive about alternative therapies—not only does it benefit the patient and keep them healthy and out of the hospital, but it benefits the insurance company as well.

The financial aspects of treatment can become very frustrating indeed; nevertheless, it is important to remember that your health is crucial and should not be overlooked.

For more information, visit "How to Price a Naturopathic Doctor" (www.ehow.com/how_2031466_price-naturopathic-doctor.html)

CHAPTER 9

Comprehensive Diet Guide for Improving Digestive Wellness

I N THIS chapter, we will provide a practical philosophy of eating that will be beneficial in living a life that is free of disease and without the aid of medications that could potentially inhibit one's quality of life. Or, the diet tips found here can be used in conjunction with a daily regimen of medications, thereby enhancing one's health and enabling the body to boost its immune function.

EACH DIET IS UNIQUE TO THE INDIVIDUAL

It is presumptuous of us to assume that one diet can be healthful and beneficial for everyone. Without taking into account one's food allergies, age, blood type, genetics, and any previous surgeries that might have hindered digestion, our diet suggestions should stand as a foundation for you to build upon for your health. We have put together the best diet possible to help the broadest population of inflammatory bowel disease patients with the idea that you will be inspired to move beyond these suggestions to discover what types of foods feel optimal for your health and what types of foods negatively impact your health.

Dede's Experience

Throughout my college years and beyond, my diet was low in fiber but high in table sugar and acidic foods. Fried foods, coffee, cigarettes, and years of improper eating habits due to a pernicious denial of food-as-pleasure lead to bulimia and irregular periods. I often had a low-grade fever and bouts of diarrhea, gas, and a swollen belly. By eating very little, I was able to keep my distended belly from looking too obvious, but the accompanying depression and anemia was harder to hide. I remember being told a few weeks before my wedding, "You look gorgeous, you look like a skeleton!" That, for me, was a wake-up call: why would 'looking like a skeleton' be considered gorgeous? This helped me realize just how confused our culture (in the United States in particular) is about beauty and thinness.

When painful ulcers form in areas of the small and large intestine, which is the case in Crohn's and colitis, the delicate balance of good and bad bacteria is disrupted. Food has trouble moving down the colon. In my case, the lack of fiber was really a problem, and I was frequently constipated; not only that, but scarring ensued after the ulcers would heal. This vicious cycle kept repeating itself, and after years of neglect, I had the adverse affect of constipation so painful at times that I couldn't drive my car to pick up the kids at school. Poor absorption of nutrients was yet another bi-product of IBD, and my hair, my nails, and my skin all had problems and lacked shine. My energy fluctuated, and I did have periods when I remained in remission. But over time, I got progressively worse.

THE BASICS: PROPER DIGESTION

Proper digestion and absorption are extremely important in overall health. Proper digestion of foods is important because the breaking down of food decreases the food particle size so that nutrients, amino acids, and fats can be taken from the food and absorbed to be utilized by the body. If digestion is altered, decreased nutrient absorption can cause significant vitamin deficiencies, which can relate to various illnesses. Also, prolonged use of NSAIDs can result in larger food particles in the intestine and, when not properly broken down, can cause problems such as arthritis.

Contributing to proper digestion are digestive enzymes and stomach acid, bile, and probiotics in the presence of controlled inflammation. Enzymes help to drive reactions that break down specific types of foods. For example, amylase helps to break down starch and lipase helps to break down lipids. Bile also plays an important part in digestion of fats and is secreted from the liver into the intestine when needed. Fat digestion and assimilation is important because fats make up cell membranes; therefore, they play a large role in making new cells within the body. HCl is present in the stomach to aid in the breakdown of proteins. Amino acids, the building blocks of proteins, are used in the body to make new proteins and act as coenzymes to help drive many metabolic reactions, making them vital for survival.

Individuals with low HCl, deficiency of pancreatic enzymes, or have had their gall bladder removed are at risk of deficient nutrient absorption. This is important because our gastrointestinal tract is like the fuel tank of a car. If it can't get the nutrients that it needs from the GI tract, it doesn't function optimally and disease can result. Supplementations with HCl, pancreatic enzymes, and bile can be extremely helpful in individuals who lack these important digestive components.

EATING A HEALTHY DIET

The very first change that should occur in patients wanting to improve their health is a dietary change! Even minor dietary changes can affect health significantly and usually larger dietary changes can bring even better results. Diet is extremely important to health. As of 2004, according to the CDC, at least ⅓ of all United States deaths were related to poor diet and lack of physical activity.[1] It is probable that deaths due to poor diet and lack of physical activity have only increased. Newer research directly relates cancer risk with poor diet and found that obesity directly increases cancer risk for various types of cancers.[2]

DIET AND INFLAMMATION

According to a recent article in *GUT*, and as reported by Anne Harding of Reuters Health (December 2, 2009), "there's currently no proven dietary treatment for ulcerative colitis, [Dr. Andrew] Hart noted, but the current findings raise the possibility that eating a diet low in linoleic acid could be helpful. While a Western-style, red-meat-heavy diet is high in this fatty acid and low in omega-3s, Hart noted, a more Mediterranean style eating pattern—with plenty of fruits and vegetables, fish, and nut oils—would be low in linoleic acid and high in omega-3."

The first step in changing your diet is to understand what types of changes you must make and imaging how you are going to implement them. If you can't see yourself doing the diet, then it will not happen. The stricter you are in the beginning, the easier it is. Once you make the diet change and are seeing your health improving and symptoms are relieved, then the diet should not have to be as strict. The key here is that your symptoms are relieved and your body has moved to a better state of wellness. If this is so, and your digestive health has improved, then you should be able to tolerate more foods. A patient might make it a rule to do really well with his diet at home but relax the rules a little at a restaurant or friend's house. Of course, this shouldn't become a habit! Eating and changing the diet this way eliminates many binging problems associated with ultra strict diets that cannot be maintained long term.

Decide what dietary changes you are going to make and begin making a plan of action for changing such as ridding your cupboards and refrigerator of unhealthy items such as white flour, white sugar, etc.

Dede's Experience: My Diet

Breakfast: Oatmeal (instant, or steel cut oats if time allows) topped with canola margarine, sliced almonds, raisins, cranberries, and dried cherries or dried blueberries, along with hot black tea with honey and milk

Mid-morning snack: 1 hard-boiled egg or 1 banana

Lunch: Homemade soup (usually vegetarian) or a salad with tuna fish or chicken salad

Mid-afternoon snack: Handful of almonds and raisins, or carrots and humus

Before dinner: Carrots or some sliced cheese with rice crackers

Dinner: Steamed vegetables and rice with baked fish

Other snacks during the day: Apples or pears (I eat whatever is local and in season)

Water: Drink as much as you can (green tea is also a great alternative if you're getting tired of drinking so much water, though it is usually caffeinated)

Before bed: Sleepytime Tea (it has valerian in it which is very relaxing), daily vitamins and supplements (Omega-3 fish oil capsules, cod liver oil, multi-vitamin without iron, magnesium, primrose oil to help with dry skin, vitamin C with garlic to help prevent flu, ground flax seed and ¼ teaspoon of "Ultra Flora Plus" probiotics, along with 1 tablespoon of a "hormone-balance" herbal tincture that my naturopath makes up for me every few months)

If I am having flare-ups, my naturopath will add other supplements such as digestive enzymes, and I occasionally use the UNDA drops (see page 118 for more information). If I am constipated, which has been a problem for me in the past, I drink the "Smooth Move" tea (made by the company Traditional Medicinals), and I also increase my exercise, get more sleep, and do more yoga and meditation.

CREATIVE DIET STRATEGIES

Eating healthily and happily involves an investment of time and creativity. Preparation helps make the diet transition go smoothly. There are many techniques to create fast, easy, and healthy meals. For example, have a raw night of hummus, veggies and crackers. Other mornings, make a green drink to start the day right with a good serving of vegetables. To create healthy meals, use techniques such as steaming, sautéing, puréeing, chopping small, blending, grinding, and many others. If you have a health food store near you or a restaurant that serves healthy meals, go there often at first and get food ideas. Looking through the deli cases at the salads can give you great ideas on how to create salads from ingredients you have at home.

Eating healthy also doesn't have to be boring. Spice up salads with nuts, seeds, veggies, and fruits. Cook whole grains and mix them with greens and fruit to make beautiful cold salads. Consider sautéing fruit with your vegetables to make a special dinner treat. Here are a few tricks.

- Use ground oats for oat flour. Use gluten-free oats if there is sensitivity to gluten. Oats can be ground simply in your coffee grinder or a high powered blender. Fresh oat flour can be used for baking, thickening soups, and thickening gravies.
- Sprinkle nuts or seeds over your stir-fries for extra protein. If you are unable to tolerate seeds whole due to risk of diverticulitis, there is no need for you to go without their extreme value. Grind the nuts and seeds to a powder in your coffee grinder and continue to add them to your meals. They offer a wholesome nutty taste.
- Grind carrots or celery into salads such as egg salad or salmon salad.
- Add nutritional yeast flakes for seasoning to almost anything including popcorn, pizza, pasta, stir-fries, and much more.
- Add antioxidant berries to cereals, oatmeals, smoothies, and sweet treats.
- Steam sweet potatoes and add them to pasta sauce.
- Add spinach to smoothies.
- Make a good vegetable soup and blend it. Use this blending mixture to cook your rice with and you make very tasty but very nutritious rice.
- Always experiment. If you can't tolerate something in a recipe, use something else. If you react to some spices, find ones that you do well with.
- Cook or bake with friends for inspiration. Have potlucks with food items that are safe for IBD or meet ahead of time to discuss ingredients that should be avoided by the group.

- Use non-gluten options for breading foods and making crusts such as corn flakes if tolerated, ground nuts and seeds, lightly ground oats, or ground crispy rice cereal.

Diet Strategies for Sensitive Digestion

No one diet is completely right for everyone with inflammatory bowel disease. Keep a food diary to find out which foods cause problems for you. Then you can avoid those foods and choose others that supply the same nutrients. Some people with IBD may have problems digesting legumes, fiber-rich foods, raw salads, spices, additives, preservatives, fried foods, and there may be others.

For those individuals who either are still having significant symptoms or have very sensitive digestion, steaming or cooking most foods, even fruits, can help significantly. By steaming or cooking most foods, it reduces the live enzyme content of the food and makes it significantly easier on your digestion if you are suffering.

Make sure to chew foods well and eat slowly. For some, taking 2 teaspoons of organic apple cider vinegar in a little bit of water before meals can aid digestion. If this is too much, reduce the amount and work up to the 2 teaspoons Bitters are also very helpful to use prior to or after meals to help with digestive ability. Bitters help by increasing gastric secreting of enzymes and HCL, which facilitate digestion. By activating gastric secretion of HCL and other digestive enzymes, the nerve stimulation to the muscles of the entire digestive tract improves. By increased nervous system stimulation and muscle movement, blood circulation improves and the body can assimilate foods, absorb nutrients, and eliminate wastes more efficiently. Bitters will be discussed further in the treatment section.

For individuals who do not know what they react to, eliminate and challenge foods to figure out your intolerances. It is best to start with a very limited anti-inflammatory and hypoallergenic diet for 4–7 weeks. After this time, then slowly add back in foods and watch for reactions. Wait three days after introducing one food before trying another to be sure of your reaction. Do this again when introducing raw foods back into the diet if you have been eating most of your foods lightly steamed or cooked.

Sometimes inflammatory bowel disease sufferers who suffer from gas, diarrhea, constipation and other ailments who have tried high fiber diets and failed, may want to try a low fiber diet initially while inflammation is being treated and reduced. This low-fiber diet can still provide nutrients and will only avoid the most troublesome fiber. During this time, nutrient supplementation will become important and can sometimes be via IV if nutritional deficiencies are largely apparent. See future section on nutrient IV replacements.

Low fiber doesn't mean that vegetables need be omitted from the diet. Make sure to include vegetable juices without pulp, potatoes without skin, alfalfa sprouts, beets, green/yellow beans, carrots, celery, cucumber without the peel, eggplant if it doesn't cause reactions, lettuce, mushrooms, green/red peppers, squash, and zucchini. Many grains can be omitted for now considering they add to the fiber load and also are acidic for the system. Avoid vegetables from the cruciferous family such as broccoli, cauliflower, brussels sprouts, cabbage, and kale, Swiss chard, etc. Clean proteins are acceptable such as chicken, turkey, fish, and eggs. Avoid all nuts and seeds unless they are ground into butters. A small amount of rice should be okay as long as it doesn't worsen symptoms. Include some fruits in your diet such as apples as long as they are in a sauce form or steamed until soft and tender, apricots, bananas, cantaloupe, grapes, honeydew melon, peaches, and watermelon. Avoid dried fruits and raw fruits except bananas. Filtered water is extremely important if you are in this stage, as it will keep everything moving in the body. Drink at least 8–10 glasses of filtered water daily.

Smoothies are an excellent way to keep nutrition up while using a low fiber diet until gastrointestinal inflammation decreases. Alternative milks in addition to coconut milk can be used with fruits, vegetables, nut butters, filtered water, and a small amount of juice to make calorie-dense, nutrient-packed snacks or meals.

This low fiber diet is not ideal for long-term use and assuming inflammation within the gastrointestinal track and the immune system imbalance is being treated, then consuming fiber may resume once gastrointestinal symptoms improve. The introduction of fiber-rich foods should be on a trial basis when initially introducing them back into the diet.

FOODS AND SPICES THAT HELP HEAL INFLAMED TISSUES

It is easy and difficult at the same time to eat healthily. It is very easy to think about changing your diet and eating healthier, but is sometimes hard to implement, especially if you have an opposing family member in your home who will not help and support your diet change.

Let's talk about foods that should be included that are either important in keeping inflammation under control in the body or offering nutrients important for optimal health and organ function. All of the following foods should be considered when developing a healthy diet regimen: fish, all vegetables except those listed on page 172, all fruits except dried and those mentioned above, nuts, seeds, and berries.

Essential fatty acids become very important to include in the diet due to their response in the inflammatory cascade. Omega 3 fatty acids have been shown to decrease overall body inflammation in many studies and help to improve lipid profiles.[3, 4] Various other studies have shown the consumption of omega 3 fatty acids to be related to symptom improvement in inflammatory bowel disease.

Omega 3 fatty acids are found in cold-water fish and fish oil, algae, walnuts, leafy green vegetables, and flax seeds. Examples of cold water fish that can be safely consumed often include mackerel, lake trout, herring, sardines, and wild salmon. The Environmental Working Group released a study on farmed salmon that revealed the content of PCB chemical found in farmed salmon exceeded the Environmental Protection Agency's limits. PCBs are cancer-causing chemicals that were banned in the United States in 1976, but continue to be present in our environment. Tests of farmed salmon purchased in U.S. grocery stores showed that, on average, farmed salmon have 16 times the amount of PCBs found in wild salmon. Omega 3 fatty acids can also be found in lower quantities in walnuts, flax seeds, and soybeans and the oils made from them, those this omega 3 fatty acid provides much less potent effects.

The Food and Drug Administration advises pregnant women to not consume shark, swordfish, king mackerel and tilefish due to their high mercury content. Everyone should avoid these high mercury fish due to mercury's potentially detrimental effect on the nervous system. The FDA does not list tuna on this dangerous list but experts suggest[5] all pregnant women, infants, children, and women of childbearing age should avoid white tuna because of its high mercury content. Use canned wild salmon instead of tuna and limit your exposure to tuna to rare restaurant experiences. Examples of algae that contain essential fatty acids and provide beneficial health effects are spirulina and chlorella. These can be used as nutritional powders and can be added to various foods for their health benefit. Both spirulina and chlorella can be found in health food stores, most likely as a capsule, but occasionally as a powder.

Other nutritional powders are also abundant and easy to find. Adding them to the diet can be very effective in helping to support proper organ and gland function. These nutritional powders consist of kelp, protein powders, brewer's yeast, ground nuts and seeds, acidophilus, acai powder, green tea powder, greens powder, slippery elm powder, ground milk thistle seeds, and hydrastis powder. These are only some of the valuable powders that you could use, but the point is to begin experimenting with adding these immensely healthy powders to your diet daily. There will be more on this in the dietary implementation section.

Add anti-inflammatory spices to every meal such as turmeric, ginger, garlic, cinnamon, rosemary, basil, cilantro, cardamom, and parsley. All of these herbs are anti-inflammatory in nature and can help to soothe the irritation within the gastrointestinal tract. If you are unsure of how to use spices in your cooking, search recipes online and be creative. All you have to do is search "turmeric chicken recipe" if you want to make a turmeric chicken. Most often, you will find the recipe you want when searching this way. Searching recipe ideas on the internet is very easy and most of the time you can find what you want to make. The more often you incorporate healthy spices into your diet, the more health benefits you will receive from them. Try the following version of Chai without black tea. This is a great recipe for people of all ages.

Chai Spiced Milk

> 1 cup filtered water
> 2 cups unsweetened rice, soy, almond, or hemp milk
> Honey or agave syrup to taste
> 1–2 teaspoon spice mixture

Mix together the following spices to make your spice mix:
> 2 parts cardomom
> 2 parts cloves
> 1 part black pepper
> 2 parts cinnamon

Then bring 1 cup of filtered water to a boil in a saucepan. Add 1–2 teaspoons of the spice mixture and 1 teaspoon fresh minced ginger and boil gently for 1 minute. Reduce heat, add two cups of unsweetened rice, almond, soy, or hemp milk. Sweeten to taste, strain through fine tea strainer or cheese cloth and enjoy warm.

THE BENEFIT OF FERMENTED FOODS

Fermented foods have enjoyed an increased awareness in recent years. The fermentation of foods and drinks has occurred in many cultures throughout the world for many years. It seems to go in and out of popularity. A recent trend towards fermented foods has occurred mostly out of our realization that cultures that consume fermented foods regularly have enjoyed a lower morbidity rate for some chronic illnesses. Fermented foods naturally have a complex balance of microorganisms that may be beneficial to the gastrointestinal lining, other mucus membrane linings within the body, and can help to balance the overall balance of microorganisms that exist on our entire body including our skin. Balancing our relationship with our symbiotic microorganisms, because they outnumber our own cells significantly, is important to the functioning of our defense systems.

Here are some examples of fermented foods: dairy kefir, juice kefir, sauerkraut, kimchee, kombucha, tempeh, and soy sauce. The Cookbook, *Nourishing Traditions* by Sally Fallon and Mary G. Enig has many fermenting ideas and recipes to get you started. The *Body Ecology Diet* by Donna Gates and Linda Schatz may also be helpful.

FOODS TO AVOID

Please see previous chapter. Foods that commonly cause reactions in individuals suffering from inflammatory conditions are listed in the table below.

Potentially Problematic Foods to Avoid	Foods and Spices to Include
Wheat or maybe ALL gluten	Cold water fish
Dairy	Nuts and seeds if tolerated
Sugar	8–10 glasses of filtered water daily
Potatoes	Fiber after disease is managed
Eggplant	Flax seed or walnut oil in salads
Tomatoes	Lean hormone-free meat
Peppers	Hormone-free eggs
Paprika	Vegetables: steamed if sensitive digestion
Cayenne	Fruits: steamed if sensitive digestion
Fiber in early stages of disease	Nutrional powders
Caffeine	Tumeric
Chocolate	Ginger
Alcohol	Rosemary
Carbonated drinks and soda	Garlic and garlic powder
Artificial sweeteners	Cinnamon
Artificial additives and preservatives	Cilantro
Fried foods	Parsley
Dried fruit	Basil
Limit gas-producing foods such as cabbage-family vegetables (broccoli, cabbage, cauliflower and Brussels sprouts), legumes, onions and chives	

PROPER MEALTIME HABITS

Proper mealtime habits should include being relaxed while eating, and ensuring proper digestion by chewing. Digestion does begin in the mouth and as we chew, we secrete saliva that begins to break down our foods and begin the digestion process. Make sure there is no TV in the background, no computers, avoid using the phone, and absolutely no eating and driving!

CHAPTER 10

Lifestyle Guide for Reducing Inflammation and Promoting Digestive Health

I N THIS chapter, you will find information on simple and inexpensive at-home therapies and lifestyle changes. Never underestimate the value of these simple therapies—particularly for patients who cannot spend a lot of money on supplements, these treatments can become invaluable.

Changing your lifestyle can be liberating and engaging. It allows one to become more aware of their body and changes that are occurring, as opposed to merely taking a drug and waiting for the symptom to disappear. Integrating whole-body treatment and lifestyle changes can help to improve overall health rather than focusing on one issue or one specific problem.

PHYSICAL TECHNIQUES THAT PROMOTE HEALTH
Rhythm Practices: Daily Prevention Tapping and Hydrotherapy

Hydrotherapy can be found in literature dating back to 5th century, B.C. by the Greek physician Hippocrates. It has since been used in many forms by physicians and laypeople all around the world.

Here are a series of simple daily routines you can do to help enhance your healing and promote better response to therapies. Many patients utilize these techniques and find they increase their connection to themselves and to their health. A part of the disease etiology for some people is our disconnection to our bodies and to our illness.

The hydrotherapy can be done first thing every morning during your regular shower. The tapping, cross crawl, and deep breathing that will be described following can either be done immediately after your shower or can be performed nearly anywhere and only require about 3 ½–4 minutes to complete. This short routine can refresh you when you are feeling tired, help you focus when you are feeling a mental block, and can help reduce stress.

PERSONAL TIP FROM DR. BLACK

I use hydrotherapy if either of my daughters seems out of sorts or has a fever, and it works every time. I also tap up and down their spines a few times before and after the treatment. I believe this helps to increase circulation to all organs by promoting nerve circulation. Now, if they are feeling particularly stressed, they often come and ask me to do the tapping for them, knowing they will feel better afterwards.

Hydrotherapy

Hydrotherapy is an excellent way to promote blood flow. Proper blood flow is needed to carry away waste and provide the necessary nutrients for organs and tissues. This can be accomplished through hot/cold showers and should be done daily. It's best to do this in the morning prior to the tapping exercises.

Hot and cold shower:

1–3 minutes hot water followed by 30 seconds cool to cold water. Repeat this sequence 3 times making sure to end on cold. Ending on cold is essential to cleansing as it brings blood back into your vital organs.

Constitutional Hydrotherapy for Colon Health

Constitutional hydrotherapy can be used for various health conditions, especially when individuals are chronically ill, have a fever or upper respiratory illness, or simply want to improve the circulation of their blood and lymphatic fluid. Try this treatment for any acute illness when a fever is present, especially in children. It is easy to perform, requires few supplies, and can be a very cost-effective way to improve overall health.

Supplies:
    4 hand towels
    2 wool, fleece or synthetic blankets

Directions:
1. Make sure the patient is warm.
2. If the patient isn't warm, apply two hot towels to the chest extending from the chest to the abdomen (covering from the neck to the pubic bone) or have them take a warm bath, but no longer than 15 minutes. Oftentimes, this step can be skipped unless the patient is experiencing chills.
3. Wring out under hot water two hot towels and apply to chest and abdomen, from the neck to the pubic bone. The towels should be as hot as the patient can tolerate and not dripping when applied to the body. Cover completely from neck to toe with 2 wool, fleece, or synthetic blankets. Make sure the patient's feet and arms are inside the blankets. Leave these two layers on for 5 minutes.

4. After 5 minutes, replace the two hot towels with the newly hot towel. Cover the patient back up while preparing the cold towel. Prepare the cold towel by running it under cold water from the faucet and wringing out completely so it is not dripping. When the cold towel is ready, replace the newly warmed towel with the cold towel. Cover patient and leave the cold towel on for 10 minutes. Most individuals will feel very warm within a few minutes of this towel. If children or babies cry or complain, most likely they will settle down within less than 1 minute and if they are ill, most will fall asleep during the cold. Make sure to reassure and hold babies to keep them comfortable.

5. Turn the patient over and repeat the sequence on the back. For infants and children, do not flip over; continue another sequence on the front.

To recap the treatment:
1. Two hot towels to chest for 5 minutes.
2. 1 hot towel immediately followed by 1 cold towel to chest for 10 minutes.
3. Flip patient over (for adults).
4. Two hot towels to the back for 5 minutes.
5. 1 hot towel immediately followed by 1 cold towel to back for 10 minutes.

Castor Oil Packs

Castor oil packs have been shown to be effective in treating some inflammatory bowel disease disorders. Castor oil, long known by many as an oral treatment for quick constipation relief, has been used for many years and is FDA approved for oral consumption in treating constipation. Most individuals who have taken castor oil orally will note its distinct taste and texture.

Castor oil is high in an unsaturated fat called ricinoleic acid. Richinoleic acid has been shown to have antimicrobial and antifungal properties; it is also known to kill molds. Interestingly enough, castor oil packs have also been shown to strengthen the immune system and stimulate an increase in white blood cells.

A stated concern in the use of castor oil is ricen. Ricen is a potentially very toxic chemical found in the castor bean. When castor oil is extracted from the castor bean, ricen is the toxic waste byproduct. It can be lethal to humans in very small quantities, although there has not yet been any ricen poisoning reported from the use of castor oil packs or using castor oil topically.

How to do a Castor Oil Pack

Castor oil applied to the skin over the liver and abdomen enhances circulation, lymph flow, detoxification and elimination—all of which help relieve symptoms of IBD. There are many applications for the use of castor oil packs including premenstrual syndrome, uterine fibroids, ovarian cysts, headaches, constipation, intestinal disorders, gallbladder, liver conditions, high blood pressure, cancer, and much more. Castor oil can also be used topically to help absorption of topical medicines. For example, it can be mixed with essential oils to facilitate their absorption into deeper layers of the mucosa for enhanced results.

Contraindications: Do not use castor oil packs with heat over uterine growths, in pregnancy, if you have ulcers, or while menstruating. Do not use an electric heating pad.

Dede's Experience

I use castor oil packs frequently even now that I am in remission. It is an easy routine to follow, though somewhat
messy. I combine my pack with plastic wrap and a dish
towel to keep the area from getting sticky, and I put it
right over my abdomen while I lay on top of my bed. I
use the pack to decrease my stress levels—just lying on the
bed and practicing relaxation techniques is quieting—and
reduce inflammation. It really works!

Supplies:

Cold pressed castor oil (available at health food stores)

Non-dyed flannel cloth (double to triple thickness) large enough
to cover from the top of your hip bones to the bottom of
your ribs

A large freezer bag for storage

Old tee-shirt or pajama top

Plastic wrap or kitchen sized plastic bag

Hot water bottle or heating pad (non-electric is preferred)

Directions:

1. Fold the flannel so that there are two to three layers of cloth.
It should be big enough to cover your abdomen and liver area
from the end of your rib cages all the way to your hipbones.

2. Saturate the flannel with castor oil so that it is soaked through,
but not dripping.

3. Lie down and place the newly saturated flannel on your abdomen, covering your liver area.

4. Place plastic (preferably a kitchen-sized garbage bag) over the
flannel and then apply the heat source. The plastic simply keeps

the castor oil from getting all over your clothes and your heating source.

5. Relax for at least 30 minutes. The best time to do this is at night before bed. This is also a good time to do visualization exercises and to focus on deep abdominal breathing.

6. Store flannel pack in glass container or plastic bag in the refrigerator or freezer. The same pack may be used for months.

Enemas

Enemas should only be used sparingly and in small quantities. There is no need to flush the colon with an overwhelming amount of solution. Instead of an enema bag, try using a syringe with a small tube on the end for introducing the solution into the rectum. That way, the solution can be pushed in gently and the amount can be measured on the syringe. Start with 5 cc and build up from there if you feel you need more of a cleanse. For babies, only if needed for constipation, use 1 cc of warm water—this usually does the trick within a day or two. For some patients suffering from inflammatory bowel conditions who are destined for surgery, enemas can provide some quicker relief and quicker results when first under natural and/or allopathic treatment.

Coffee enemas are used to help stimulate the liver to flush by increasing bile production. This can be helpful in a patient who is overly burdened by emotional or physical stress, on multiple medications, has had a history of improper bowel function, or has a strong history of chemical exposure. Coffee enemas do not heal the tissue in inflammatory bowel disease; they merely stimulate the liver and begin the detoxification process. These could be used first if the colon is not extremely inflamed or has fissures. Only freshly brewed organic coffee should be used, not instant coffee. Don't use the coffee if the solution is too hot.

If the colon is inflamed, coffee enemas are not recommended because the gastrointestinal tract lining needs to heal first. Herbal enemas can be very soothing if there is irritated tissue, fissures, and large amounts of inflammation.

Here are a few herbs used for making healing enema teas:

- marshmallow root
- cayenne (safe for intestinal bleeding)
- comfrey root
- calendula
- aloe
- catnip
- slippery elm (helps to coat and soothe the gastrointestinal lining and can also help treat diarrhea)

If there are parasites, yeast, or bacterial overgrowth in the gastrointestinal lining, then garlic enemas may be used to kill the offending organism while systemic treatment commences.

Soothing Suppositories

Suppositories can be very helpful and somewhat easier to use than enemas. They can be created by a naturopathic physician to contain the appropriate balance of healing and soothing components for improving colon function and reducing inflammation. These suppositories may contain vitamin A, vitamin E, and other herbal compounds including some of the ones listed in Chapter 8: Treatment Options.

Suppositories used by allopathic physicians (such as Entocort, which contains budenoside, a compound that is similar to prednisone but with less systemic activity) can be extremely helpful in reducing flare-ups or beginning the initial healing process by decreasing inflammation. Mesalamine enemas or suppositories may also be prescribed by an allopathic physician depending on the site of damage or inflammation within the intestine. Though these treatments are not always the best choice, sometimes they are needed if inflammation and/or bleeding are severe.

Dede's Experience

When I was first hospitalized in 2001, my stepsister very kindly offered me the name of her 'energy medicine' coach, and I was immediately skeptical. Terms like "chakras" and "intuitive wellness" were just not a part of my vocabulary. The nature of my disease, intestinal scarring due to flare-ups and inflammation, was something tangible, and I wondered how it could possibly be treated with spiritual guidance or ethereal dialogue from an intuitive wellness practitioner. Thus my doubts initially overruled any desire to contact this "coach." The other factor was cost—I worried that these coaches were not in my budget, and at first I felt I couldn't really justify it as a legitimate "out of pocket medical expense."

When I had my recurrence and was hospitalized, I made an appointment with the surgeon in order to better understand what was going to happen during my upcoming bowel resection. I began to think that it might not be a bad idea to "cover my bases" and consult with an energy medicine therapist to help alleviate my fears.

I called Laura Alden Kamm, the spiritual energy medicine therapist whose name had been given to me. Laura Alden Kamm had written a book I read the month before my surgery entitled *Intuitive Wellness*. I read the book cover-to-cover, just as I had read many other books during that time of uncertainty. I was skeptical of Laura's book from the onset, due to my own inhibitions, but once I started reading it, I couldn't put it down.

For my session with Laura, we had a prearranged time, and a pre-paid credit card transaction via the internet. I called a number she gave me and she answered right away.

Being somewhat nervous, uptight, and skeptical, I asked her how she worked. "Vibrations," was her reply. She said she sat in a room with gray walls and no distractions and actually felt the vibrations coming from me, my voice, and my energy, as I talked to her over the phone.

A skeptical reader may wonder if I was the victim of a hoax, as I did initially, but I began to "let go" of my fears as I listened to Laura's soothing voice. Having read her book and her own account of her near-death experience, I knew that she had devoted her life to helping others open themselves up to healing with generally positive results and much-improved health and well-being amongst her clients.

I became one of those clients, and working with Laura really gave me confidence to heal.

After the session with Laura, I had this pronounced feeling of utter calm and confidence that not only had the surgery worked, but that I had an active role in making it work and keeping the disease at bay from the very real threat of recurrence.

As an aside, Laura also gently and intuitively noted that my father was sick with cancer, and she knew that this was going to be hard for me going forward with my own healing journey. Sadly, my father died just over a year after my surgery, but in a small way, I was better prepared for his passing having had some coaching from Laura beforehand.

We ended the session with her sending me a recorded CD so I could listen and practice some of the exercises she recommended, like Spinal Chakra Breathing. Nowadays, Laura can email an MP3 instead, and the patient can listen to the session and practice some of her meditations. To this day, I use the Spinal Chakra Breathing to help alleviate stress.

Tapping for Energy

This tapping technique was modified from *Energy Medicine* from Donna Eden.[1] It is a great book to reference if you feel confident doing the tapping and want to do more complex tapping routines daily. Daily tapping is very energy focused and effective.

This tapping procedure involves tapping on five areas within the body that serve as acupuncture meridian points which increase the flow of energy, or life force, that flows through these associated organs daily. Doing this tapping daily keeps the energy flowing and increases circulation, which helps reduce disease.

According to Henry Lindlar, M.D., who was diagnosed with diabetes in the 1900s, often disease and illness arise from the inadequate circulation and nutrient content of the blood and lymphatic fluid. We know this to be true because we often see patients' symptoms diminish as they improve their circulation and nutrient exchange through proper nutrient intake, proper absorption, and exercise and movement therapies. Even medicines work better if patients are regularly eliminating properly, eating properly, exercising, and drinking filtered water.

The diagram on page 186 lists the five points you will tap daily as part of your daily prevention tapping. Each area should be lightly tapped repetitively for thirty seconds. Tapping these areas daily should increase energy, stimulate immune function, increase concentration, and increase strength and vitality.

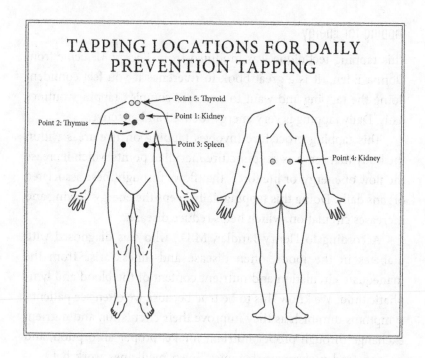

TAPPING LOCATIONS FOR DAILY PREVENTION TAPPING

Point 5: Thyroid
Point 1: Kidney
Point 2: Thymus
Point 3: Spleen
Point 4: Kidney

1. Kidney point: Put fingers on your clavicle; run them midline until you can feel the larger bumps at the proximal end of your clavicle. Drop your fingers about an inch lower and slightly outward.
2. Thymus point: Move your fingers midline and down 2 inches to the center of your sternum.
3. Spleen points: Located at the rib line directly under each nipple, bilaterally.
4. Adrenal/kidney: Located in the middle back (one on each side of the spine), you can turn your hands inward and use the thumb side and back of your hands bilaterally.
5. Thyroid: Located over the Adam's apple area.

Cross Crawl for Balanced Thought and Improved Focus

The cross crawl is an exaggerated march which was developed by studying what our body normally does when it is physically active. By utilizing opposite sides of the body to perform a repetitive motion, it stimulates a better connection and communication from the left side of the brain to the right. This can improve focus, balance, clarity, and overall metabolism. It also increases energy and enhances breathing and stamina.

It is performed by standing in a comfortable spot on the floor with enough room to raise your arms and legs. Obese, wheel chair bound, or persons with poor balance can remain seated and either lift their arms and legs or only move their arms if unable to move their legs.

The cross crawl should be performed daily, and especially prior to taking tests, going to work or school, or any other time when your mind needs to remain sharp.

To do the cross crawl:

1. Lift your right arm and left leg at the same time.
2. As you let your arm and leg down, then lift your left arm and right leg at the same time.
3. Continue an exaggerated march in this fashion for at least one minute, breathing deeply in through your nose and out through your mouth.

Deep Breathing

Making sure to breathe deeply is important for your health. Deep breathing exercises are extremely effective in handling depression, anxiety, and stress-related disorders.

Begin by inhaling through the nose as much as you can, paying attention to the abdomen and making sure it is freely moving and expanding to allow air in. Breathe out through the mouth and begin again with the next deep breath. Do this for at least five complete breaths. If you have time for more, continue this for another minute or so.

> Doing these daily prevention techniques and making them habit is the first step in building an exercise program, if you are not already doing so. You will likely notice a difference fairly quickly after adopting this program daily.
>
> Don't knock it until you try it. The next time you are feeling fatigued or down, force yourself to do a routine that involves the tapping, followed by the cross crawl, followed by the breathing, and notice how energized you become!

Exercise

Exercise is one of the most important lifestyle practices to adopt when considering treatment options. No matter what your physical state is, there is always something you can do for exercise. If you currently do not have an exercise routine, are dangerously overweight, or have had a hard time sticking to an exercise program in the past, begin by mastering the daily prevention techniques described earlier in this chapter. Once you are doing those daily and feel you can proceed onto a more formal form of exercise, be sure to explore all of your options to find the best one for you.

Here are some examples:
1. Running in place
2. Cross crawl (see page 187)
3. Using a hula hoop
4. Jumping rope

5. Walking with intervals of increased speed
6. Running
7. Elliptical routine
8. Weight lifting
9. Hiking
10. Swimming
11. Biking or stationary biking
12. Rebounding
13. Dancing
14. Yoga
15. Qigong
16. Tai Chi
17. Pilates

Exercise is most effective when it is performed consistently. Therefore, you should choose a few of options and make sure you are doing something almost daily. For example, if you choose an elliptical machine at the gym and work out for 45–60 minutes but can only make it to the gym 3 days per week, then you should choose another activity such as the cross crawl and make sure to do that at least 5–10 minutes on the days you don't exercise. This way, even on the days that you are not doing a work out, you are still moving and ensuring improved circulation in the body.

Implementing exercise into your schedule can be difficult if you don't already do it regularly. The best way to resolve this is to schedule exercise into your schedule. Pick a realistic time that you can be consistent with and begin immediately. You do not have to wait until you are in shape, lose weight, or get a membership to the gym. You also don't have to spend a lot of money to implement an exercise routine. The simplest form of exercise is running or jogging in place, dancing, or the cross crawl.

Dede's Experience

Exercise should be considered mandatory for everyone. Without movement and energy being burned, the body will inevitably shut down from lack of use. A kind of stasis sets in, and it starts to affect one's health.

When I was in college, I was on the tennis team, the soccer team, and the Women's Squash Team where I competed in the NCAA—a three-season athlete (which would be impossible in today's highly competitive college sports world)!

Being a so-called "jock," I was always running, playing tennis, hiking, paddling, swimming, etc., in my later years.

Nowadays, exercise is just plain fun—as it should be! When I moved to Vermont almost 25 years ago, my next-door neighbor (a retired farmer I might add), used to scoff at me when I donned my jogging outfit and headed down the street. "What are ye doing that fer?" Mr. Miller would yell as I passed by his house, waving. It is comical to me now to remember Mr. Miller, who was wondering why someone would take time to jog when they could just work on a farm, or walk the 5 miles he had to walk to school each day. Why, in fact, was our culture so obsessed with diets and thin-ness, while people were becoming obese with each successive generation?

My maxim for exercise is simple: do it a lot, and do it every day. Obviously, when you are having a flare-up, it is hard to contemplate; but starting slowly the way I did (walking to the mailbox was my first goal) is a way to integrate movement and exercise and the natural release of beneficial brain chemicals like serotonin.

One of my favorite activities that covers my daily dose of exercise, gets my heart rate up, and builds stamina and endurance is riding my bike to work whenever weather permits. I enjoy the satisfaction of saving gas money and feeling relaxed as I pedal the 5 miles in each morning (though going home is mostly those same 5 miles going uphill, which can be a bit daunting at the end of an eight hour workday).

On weekends, a group of my friends sometimes plan to meet at 8:00 A.M. in a parking lot and we carpool to various hikes around the region, pulling back into the parking lot around noon. This type of exercise also offers a social component, which is another important part of maintaining good health—being active and social, or even getting out and doing all of the above with your children, thereby instilling in them a lifelong love of exercise and enjoyment that they will carry with them into adulthood.

MENTAL AND EMOTIONAL TECHNIQUES THAT PROMOTE HEALTH
Commitment to Heal

The emotional body is so important when conquering disease and illness and can have profound power over the physical body. Believing one is well is the first, and most important, step in healing.

Dede's Experience

Jon Kabat Zinn is the founder of the Stress Reduction Clinic at University of Massachusetts Memorial Medical Center, and Saki Santorelli is the director. Since I could not travel to attend one of their courses, I read Santorelli's book, *Heal Thy Self: Lessons on Mindfulness in Medicine*. In one of my favorite exercises from the book, you are asked to hold a few raisins in your hand and meditate on them. Many of the participants in their program at University of Massachusetts Medical Center have chronic disease, and they have never had the opportunity to slow down and meditate, as shocking as that seems; for me, I was the same way—I thought meditation was something I didn't have time to do! According to founder, Kabat Zinn, "you can't stop the waves, but you can learn to surf." He has also said,

> "Generosity is another quality which, like patience, letting go, non-judging, and trust, provides a solid foundation for mindfulness practice. You might experiment with using the cultivation of generosity as a vehicle for deep self-observation and inquiry as well as an exercise in giving. A good place to start is with yourself. See if you can give yourself gifts that may be true blessings, such as self-acceptance, or some time each day with no purpose. Practice feeling deserving enough to accept these gifts without obligation—to simply receive from yourself, and from the universe."

What I most enjoyed about reading the book and bringing mindfulness into my life on a daily basis was how to use that newfound knowledge to take more responsibility for my own health and well-being, especially in light of the complex world of chronic digestive disease that I am part of.

The "Commitment to Heal" integrates thought field therapy and biolinguistic kinesiology for a simple and easy to follow technique that can be practiced without a practitioner. If you seek more knowledge or treatment in this area, seek a practitioner who practices either thought field therapy or biolinguistic kinesiology.

Thought Field Therapy: Oftentimes we experience thought patterns that create subtle energy losses within our bodies. We use chemical messengers to mediate all body processes, including the emotions we have. For each emotion, we are using chemical messengers that stimulate particular nerve patterns. When we continually stimulate these same nerve patterns with a consistent emotion (for example, depression) our body, in a sense, gets accustomed to that emotion happening again. Just like our nerves can become addicted to exogenous chemicals such as nicotine, heroine, or caffeine, it can get addicted to an endogenous chemical repetitively used for a particular emotion.

Biolinguistic kinesiology is the process of using muscle testing and counseling to find and correct emotional, mental, or physical blockages of energy caused by deep-seated emotional issues.

The Commitment to Heal process directs the mind and subconscious to address these destructive patterns. The resulting state is one in which the patient is able to communicate his or her concern with an empowering inner state of positive thinking and agreement to heal.

For example, if a person suffers from depression constantly, then depression chemicals become a normal presence within the body. If that person were to have a day without feeling depressed, his or her body will seek that same chemical to maintain its normal state of functioning. You may have seen this in a depressed person who tends to be negative about many situations and can have a good time one minute and the next minute feel unsatisfied and unhappy. This person's body feels more balanced and within homeostasis with the depression chemicals present. Again, our bodies can get addicted to certain emotions, just as we can get addicted to nicotine, heroine, or caffeine because they are chemical responses within the body.

In the Commitment to Heal, we use positive thought patterns to stimulate more positive chemicals on a regular basis while tapping particular points within the body. The tapping points are located at particular meridian points within the body, as explained earlier in this chapter.

The first step in the Commitment to Heal is to recognize any core issues that you may have. Most people have trouble recognizing or acknowledging their core issues, but many destructive emotional patterns stem from feelings of inadequacy or worthlessness.

There are two ways to follow the Commitment to Heal. The first (and simpler) technique is to work on one single statement each morning while practicing the tapping points. The second technique is to find five core issues that you want to deal with and practice all 5 every morning.

The First Technique

If you choose to do the first technique, the sentence to start on is, "I completely love and accept myself." Oftentimes, the more uncomfortable the sentence feels to an individual, the more it is needed. Each morning, the person recites this sentence each time a different meridian is tapped. See Appendix B for a list of the tapping locations.

The Second Technique

This technique is a little more complex, but if you have the time and have some severe emotional issues that you want and need to work on, it is very effective. It is a combination of thought field therapy and biolinguistic kinesiology taught by Dr. John Dye, a naturopathic physician practicing in Arizona who also teaches at the Southwest

College of Naturopathic Medicine. See Appendix B for step-by-step instructions for this second technique in the Commitment to Heal.

Meditation

Meditation is an extremely important, yet very simple, relaxation tool. There are many different types and forms of mediation so you should familiarize yourself with meditation before trying to perform it to avoid feeling a sense of failure if you don't know how to do it or what to expect the first time.

One of the simplest forms of meditation involves paying attention to your breath. During this meditation, you should get into a comfortable sitting position and begin breathing. It is helpful to set a timer if you want or need your session to only last for a certain amount of time. This will prevent you from continually checking a clock or watch during your mediation. Preferably, you should perform this mediation in a place that there will be no distractions or interruptions. Once you are seated in a comfortable position and breathing restfully for a few minutes, begin paying close attention to your breath, particularly how it moves in and out of your lungs in a fluid and calming manner. Don't count your breaths and don't judge what you are going to get out of the meditation. In fact, don't judge anything. Just breathe and concentrate on your breath. When your mind wanders, which will happen dozens of times, simply acknowledge that your mind wandered and bring yourself back to concentrating on your breath.

Over time, this sort of meditation teaches you to trust time and space and helps you to feel more connected with your physical body. Remember, place no judgment about anything during the mediation and even if your mind wanders many times, don't judge yourself as non-successful at meditating.

Dede's Experience: My Relaxation Routine

After my surgery, I had a distended and tender, quite swollen abdomen. I could barely walk. So each day, I made a goal for myself: walk to the mailbox for the first 2 days; then walk to the stop sign in the next 3 days, etc. This really helped.

Now, I rise early every morning and follow a routine.

Beginning with the rising of the sun is helpful for patients who are recovering from surgery, or a flare-up, to slow down the pace of their lives. First, I lie in bed and just breathe. I empty my mind, reflect on any dreams and let them fade, too. Watching the sunrise, I begin to think about my day—however, first it is time to greet the day. "Sun salutations," as yogis call them, are a very beneficial way to open up the heart and mind and create a healing environment.

Before I begin my daily yoga practice, I walk the dog to the mailbox to get the paper. This has become a very symbolic ritual for me, since my surgery. Before I get to the house, I look to the East to check on the progress of the sun, or check the weather. I always think of "red sky in the morning," and take pride in the rhyme at the end, "and sailors take warning," as it reminds me of my late father—a Navy man and longtime navigator of the waters of coastal Rhode Island. Observing the sky, the leaves, the grass—our surroundings in nature—is one of the greatest gifts I have received as a person who has come out on the other side of disease. Someone once said to me, "Oh, you know about life; you, who have suffered a great deal and have been healed."

Five or six years ago, I would have thought this routine

to be mumbo jumbo; plus, I didn't have time for sunrise rambles with the dog—I had a business to run and kids to get ready for school. Now, I understand that the time I save by not rushing through my day is time I can use for shopping for fresh, organic vegetables and other ingredients for dinner, or going for a 1–2 mile walk.

Once I return from walking the dog, I make myself some tea, eat breakfast, and read the paper.

After the tea and oatmeal and a quick read of a few articles in the paper, I am ready for the next part of my ritual (and by far one of the most grounding and life-affirming things I embarked on after my crisis and surgery for Crohn's disease). I go down to the basement, where I have set up a yoga "studio" of sorts. It is primitive, but it is a "room of one's own," to paraphrase the author Virginia Woolf.

I have a nice woolen rug in front of the TV, a small "altar" that consists of a small wooden statue of the Buddha surrounded by symmetrically placed candles in handmade ceramic bowls that my friend, Christie Herbert, made for me. I also have a stick of lavender incense (for relaxing aromatherapy) nearby, a photo of my late father when he was a young man, a small row of hanging Tibetan prayer flags that were set there after he died, and a tapestry hanging behind the scene. I light candles and incense, turn on the TV and the DVD, and enjoy the soothing voice of yoga guru, Rodney Yee.

Rodney Yee's "A.M. Yoga" tape is a universally applicable entry into the basics of yoga, meditation, and relaxation that can be useful for yogis at any level or non-yogis who are stiff and out-of-shape, like I was after my surgery.

Engaging in Friendships for Emotional Support

Having a companion or someone who offers emotional support is extremely important for wellness. If you do not have a spouse, family member, or close friend, you can try the following suggestions to help increase your emotional support. If you do have a spouse or family member but your relationship is not close, you may want to consider taking steps in mending the relationship into a positive experience or seeking additional emotional support in the form of friends, neighbors, fellow patients, etc.

Activity suggestions for finding emotional support:

- Disease support groups: be sure that discussion and ideas are centered in positive thoughts and positive talk
- Diet or cooking groups/classes
- Knitting classes or groups
- Card clubs
- Exercise groups/clubs or walking groups
- Book clubs
- Volunteering regularly
    Serve food at a food bank, volunteer to teach people to read, volunteer to help build homes
    Use your skills to help others
- Make friends with neighbors, co-workers
- Arrange play dates for your children with other parents to meet them and generate friendships, if possible. After all, it is also helpful to know the parents of the children your children are spending time with.
- Join local community groups: neighborhood associations, parent teacher's associations, church groups
- Go to church or other community gatherings of faith

Dede's Experience

Once a week, I attend a yoga class at a local yoga studio where I feel comfortable and supported. My yoga teacher knows I have Crohn's disease. It is also a social outlet with a lot of laughter and sharing. Once, when I could not adequately "finish" a yoga pose, I complained aloud that I could not do it. My teacher, Elisabeth Gardner, came over and quietly said to me, "Dede, your yoga practice is your *own* yoga practice—you will learn to let your body stretch into a pose by breathing into the pose and relaxing. It is not something that is judged, or graded."

I took this advice to heart, and it has helped me immensely in my daily yoga practice, but also in my relationship to my own body, and to other people in my class. By getting out and going to a class, one is immediately put into a social situation, which is a good balance to have in life—the quiet times in nature, work, home and some outside activity.

Another, somewhat embarrassing situation (as a Crohn's patient, embarrassing situations tend to loom large in our day-to-day lives) I found myself in was when one of my yoga teachers, Peter Rizzo, came to my aid during a shoulder stand where you use the wall to help support and elongate your back. My shirt fell away from my belly a bit and I tried to pull it down to cover my scar. I told Peter I was embarrassed about my scar, and his uninhibited reply was, "your scar is so beautiful; it is part of who you are and a part of your yoga practice."

CAN LAUGHTER REALLY BE THE BEST MEDICINE?

Laughter is so important for emotional and physical health. In fact, researchers in Japan found laughter very effective in reducing inflammatory cytokines in rheumatoid arthritis patients.[2] The same cytokines that were affected in this study are irregularly elevated in inflammatory bowel disease patients. Therefore, we can make the assumption that laughter can affect inflammatory cytokines and may be an effective adjunctive therapy in the treatment of inflammatory bowel disorders.

Another study published in the *American Society of Hypertension Journal* supports that laughter coupled with yoga, which they term "laughter yoga", significantly reduced patient's diastolic and systolic blood pressure in addition to reducing patient's stress hormone, cortisol.[3] Laughter yoga sounds fun![4]

Dede's Experience

One thing that is helpful when diagnosed with a digestive disease is to look at your life and its stresses, and take stock in where you are and how you function. For me, it was work, work, work, and very little play. So, each day I try to fit in a little "play" and a time to really let loose and laugh.

LEARN BODY AWARENESS

For an entire week, try writing in a journal all the symptoms your body has and everything you are doing and eating. Be sure to record all symptoms, from the most minor crick in the neck to low back pain, to headaches, to diarrhea. By doing this, you can learn how your body is trying to communicate with you, how you can listen to your body, and then change if you need to. The more you do this, easier it will become to notice these connections.

Dede's Experience

More and more of us, especially those of us who are office workers, slouch in front of a computer all day long. We forget to walk, stretch, and our posture is always forward-bending. Stress is caught up in our body in this way.

In addition to the release of breath, part of my yoga practice, and many others' as well, is the opening up of your heart. According to the American Buddhist nun, and respected yoga teacher, Pema Chodron,

"When you begin to touch your heart or let your heart be touched, you begin to discover that it's bottomless, that it doesn't have any resolution, that this heart is huge, vast, and limitless. You begin to discover how much warmth and gentleness is there, as well as how much space."

For example, maybe you have diarrhea intermittently but can never relate it to anything. By doing the journal, you may learn that each time you have a double tall caramel macchiato, you have diarrhea 3 hours later. If you notice a connection similar to this, then you know that you should do what is right and healthy for your body and stop consuming any foods or drinks that do not agree with your body. Another example would be if you notice that you are constipated each time your period is about to begin. In this case, you may have some problems with hormone regulation and should be evaluated by a naturopathic physician to make sure your hormones and glandular function is occurring optimally.

Each of the techniques in this chapter will help you to bring awareness back to your body and, when practiced daily, can help you become more body aware and more willing to take on new lifestyle changes that will improve your health.

Dede's Experience

Now that I am in remission and utterly grateful for having my life back, I have developed a newfound appreciation for the subtle things in life—a bell chiming, the wind blowing, the smell of damp leaves. As my sister, Connie, wrote to me in an email from her home in California,

> "Even if [my sisters] Marcie, Alex, Ann and I can't physically be there, each one of us is with you every single step of the way. I sort of sense that, intuitively. Sometimes I think as we get older, the universe shrinks and intensifies in an astonishingly beautiful way, i.e., our—or at least my—

universe seems to be folding in on itself. Every time I take a hike or swim in the ocean or see my kids or think of you guys, or the leaves move in the coral tree outside my bedroom, I feel overwhelmed by these very simple, lovely sensations."

Many readers and practitioners will identify with what I like to call a "survivor mentality," which is a newfound appreciation of life. Through my yoga and meditation practice, I have gained a great release, like a long exhalation of breath that I gathered and locked up inside me.

CHAPTER 11

Putting it All Together: From Disease to Wellness

FROM DISEASE TO WELLNESS: A 3-MONTH PLAN

This plan was developed as a guide for generating a treatment regimen. Just as each individual is unique, so too is their road to wellness. This 3-month plan is meant to be used loosely, so you should feel free to adjust each step as needed for your own recovery. Please consult your physician when beginning this program, and continue to visit your established team of specialists (naturopath, gastroenterologist, etc.) so that they can help you monitor your progress and make any necessary adjustments to the program.

As discussed previously, treatments and lifestyle changes can occur in any order, but here we have provided a plan that will slowly and gently move you through your digestive problems and into wellness. Most patients will feel some positive changes as they progress through this 3-month plan and some patients may even become symptom-free.

The most important aspect of this step-by-step process for building health is that we are creating a foundation for wellness and building upon it, rather than trying to overwhelm the body by incorporating all changes at once. Taking new strides each week helps to keep you focused and motivated through the entire process. We know that change can be overwhelming, which is why we've created this program so that it can also be slowed down even further to incorporate new changes every 3 weeks and can be specifically tailored to your individual needs. See the sample implementation figure below.

All severe conditions and the need for surgery must be ruled out by your physician prior to starting this program.

If initial acute symptoms are severe, they must be treated either with natural medicine or pharmaceutical medicines to provide relief while working on the underlying imbalances. See acute treatment suggestions on page 208.

Weeks 1–2:

1. See the change and believe in the change! Visualize optimal colon health daily. See yourself happy, active, and vibrant in your mind.
2. Proper Mealtime Habits (see page 173).
3. Remove major dietary causes of inflammation (see page 62).
4. Add only one supplement or herbal medicine, whichever best suits you. This may be an acute remedy for diarrhea, acidophilus, or any other supportive medicine listed in previous chapters.
5. Herbal teas: pick one of the teas that best fit your needs and drink 3 cups daily (see page 142).

Weeks 3–4:

1. Continue previous points.
2. Add an additional supplement or herbal medicine.

3. Begin the Tapping for Energy technique or daily acupressure (see page 185).
4. Experiment with adding more anti-inflammatory foods and spices into your diet.

Weeks 5–6:

1. Continue previous points.
2. Add an additional supplement or herbal medicine.
3. Begin to incorporate movement/exercise. Do this at least 3 times per week, but daily possible.

Weeks 7–8:

1. Continue previous points.
2. Incorporate daily nutritional powders into your diet such as spirulina, kelp, green tea, or acai powder (see page 144).
3. Add an additional supplement, if needed.

Weeks 9–10:

1. Continue previous points.
2. Add an additional supplement if needed.
3. Incorporate mental and emotional support (see page 191). This may be needed sooner in some individuals suffering from anxiety and depression contributing to their illness.

Weeks 11–12:

1. Continue previous points.
2. Add an additional supplement if still needing more support.
3. Incorporate colon hydrotherapy (castor oil packs 5 days per week or constitutional hydrotherapy treatments 2–4 times per week, see page 176–178).

SAMPLE TREATMENT SUGGESTIONS FOR 3-MONTH PLAN TO WELLNESS

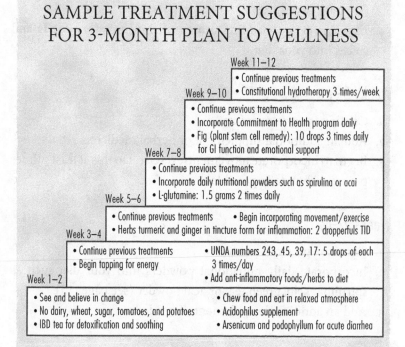

Week 11–12
- Continue previous treatments
- Constitutional hydrotherapy 3 times/week

Week 9–10
- Continue previous treatments
- Incorporate Commitment to Health program daily
- Fig (plant stem cell remedy): 10 drops 3 times daily for GI function and emotional support

Week 7–8
- Continue previous treatments
- Incorporate daily nutritional powders such as spirulina or acai
- L-glutamine: 1.5 grams 2 times daily

Week 5–6
- Continue previous treatments   • Begin incorporating movement/exercise
- Herbs turmeric and ginger in tincture form for inflammation: 2 dropperfuls TID

Week 3–4
- Continue previous treatments   • UNDA numbers 243, 45, 39, 17: 5 drops of each
- Begin tapping for energy   3 times/day
                                          • Add anti-inflammatory foods/herbs to diet

Week 1–2
- See and believe in change   • Chew food and eat in relaxed atmosphere
- No dairy, wheat, sugar, tomatoes, and potatoes   • Acidophilus supplement
- IBD tea for detoxification and soothing   • Arsenicum and podophyllum for acute diarrhea

Example of what a treatment plan may look like. Each step may be altered to fit each individual's needs.

ACTIVE DISEASE PLAN: ACUTE TREATMENT

Sometimes, a person may be in such acute distress that going into the 3-month plan for wellness may not be the best starting point. If you are extremely ill and have recurring diarrhea, fissures, or other extreme symptoms, please consult your physician to get your symptoms treated and under control before beginning the 3-month plan to wellness. Treatment of fissures to reduce bleeding and sensitivity of the rectal tissue is extremely important prior to beginning the 3-month plan to wellness. Below are some treatment ideas for acute symptoms associated with inflammatory bowel disease.

Homeopathic remedies may be useful in acute cases of diarrhea, rectal bleeding, gas, or constipation. Please see the homeopathy section on page 115.

Charcoal: If diarrhea is significant and no relief is obtained through the use of homeopathic remedies, then activated charcoal may be used. Charcoal is an excellent, easy-to-use supplement, but should only be used for a short period of time. If the need for charcoal extends past one or two weeks, consult a physician about the unrelenting diarrhea problem.

Charcoal can be used as 2–4 capsules, 3 times per day during acute diarrhea. This amounts to about 500–1000 mg., 3 times per day. Do not exceed 3 grams daily.

Herbal remedies and teas: Herbal teas effectively soothe and restore the gastrointestinal mucus membrane. If there is acute irritation, enemas and oral preparations of these teas can be used for weeks prior to starting the 3-month wellness plan. Beginning from a less inflamed state may increase effectiveness of the treatment plan, boost energy, and help to maintain motivation and a positive outlook. Please see the herbal tea and enema section on pages 142 and 181 to determine which treatment is best for you.

Suppositories for fissures: Sometimes colon inflammation is so extreme that rectal suppositories are needed. These could be herbal, compounded, or pharmaceutical and all may reduce inflammation in the colon so that you can begin the 3-month plan to wellness.

Acidophilus can be used for most acute IBD symptoms. Beginning on a high quality acidophilus prior to starting the 3-month plan to wellness will begin the healing and balancing process within the body.

MAINTENANCE PLAN

After finishing the 3-month plan to wellness, patients generally feel much better. Digestion, mood, and sleep are typically improved, and colon symptoms are decreased. At this time, you should maintain the daily regimen of treatments for at least another 6–9 months. After this time, if you continue to do well, you can consider decreasing some of the supplements but remain consistent with lifestyle changes such as diet, exercise, tapping for energy, proper dietary habits, etc.

Acidophilus can now be alternated with slippery elm powder and does not need to be taken every day. Garlic can be eaten one day per week to help kill unwanted organisms in the gastrointestinal tract.

Some other maintenance supplements that patients can take regularly to help them maintain good health are fish oil, a multivitamin, herbal teas, spices, and nutritional powders.

PART III:

Recipes for Wellness:
How to Reduce Inflammation
Through Diet

CHAPTER 12

Recipes

Ingredients: Most of the ingredients used in these recipes can be found at your local health food store or online, delivered to your home.

Microwaving food: This should be done sparingly when cooking or reheating foods because the process actually destroys important nutrients in the food.

Equipment: We suggest you keep in your kitchen a small food chopper, coffee grinder (for grinding nuts and seeds), blender or Vitamix, and non-aluminum sautéing pans.

Quality foods: Whenever possible, choose organic foods free of hormones, pesticides, and other chemicals. Buy your meats fresh or local and hormone-free, if possible. Vegetables are best when purchased fresh. A few vegetables may be purchased frozen for ease of use such as peas. Never buy canned vegetables or fruits with the exception of rare canned tomatoes, beans or canned salmon.

LOCAL, FRESH FOOD

Joining a neighborhood farm or a community supported agriculture (CSA) farm can be a great way to obtain local, fresh ingredients while also supporting family farms and reducing the use of fossil fuels to ship produce from far away. CSAs supply a group of subscribers (who pay approximately $350 or $450 per year, depending on how large a share of the vegetables they want) with a weekly allotment of veggies and root crops, as well as flowers, maple syrup, vinegars, and anything else that is in season. According to a *New York Times* article "[T]he distribution system in which people buy shares in return for a weekly allotment of local farm food has never been more popular."[1]

Joining a CSA may also encourage you to try new foods that you never would have purchased at the local supermarket.

All in all, buying fresh and local is good for the gut and the environment. Books such as *The Omnivore's Dilemma* by Michael Pollen are informative resources, and joining a community "localvore" movement are all great ways to get involved. You can even start a garden and grown your own fruits and vegetables. After all, there is nothing better than cooking together as a family, going out to your garden, to pick fresh lettuce in the summer, and making a salad while sipping some red wine.

Shopping: For those of you blessed to live in parts of the country that have easy access to healthy choices, shopping will be easy. For those of you who don't live near, or have access to, healthier food choices, shopping online can be very easy and actually cost-effective. There are many sites online from which quality food products can be purchased. Companies like Azure Standard provide fresh and shelf-stable organic products delivered right to your home or an area nearby.

This recipe section is dedicated to cooks of this century who still want to cook at home but without the complex and time-consuming processes of the past. Let's face it: it is not realistic for most families to spend hours cooking in the kitchen everyday. So, we have compiled this collection of recipes that are designed to be quick and simple while still remaining nutritiously tailored to the needs of IBD patients. We have included a few recipes for each category such as breakfasts, entrees, desserts, soups, and salads. Use what you learn from these recipes to begin developing your own. Everyone has different tastes and cultivating your palate takes time, patience, and sometimes trial and error. Learning to cook healthily is a process just like healing so keep at it and stay positive.

These recipes are meant to compliment everything you have learned thus far about how to take care of yourself and how to live easily and healthfully with inflammatory bowel disease. In fact, this section is a part of your therapy in the process of healing the inflamed bowel. Remember, what you put into the gastrointestinal tract can have a direct affect on its functioning; therefore, nurturing it with nutrient-rich, anti-inflammatory foods sets the optimal foundation for healing.

However, you should keep in mind that not all recipes work for everyone. For example, some colitis or Crohn's patients may not be able to tolerate legumes due to extreme gas. Please consider what you can and cannot tolerate when planning your meals. These recipes are suggestions; feel free to substitute ingredients for your individual needs and tastes and for those of your family.

Also see Chapter 8 (page 142) for herbal tea recipes.

COOKING TO AID HEALING

When your body is healing, it needs easily digestible, nutritious foods to aid in the process. Choice ingredients, adequate cooking, and then blending meet this need. Additionally, the healing process requires adequate nutrients, especially easily digested protein. There is often inflammation associated with illness and/or recovery, and so the anti inflammatory foods reduce swelling and inflammation and speed recovery. Enzymes are important to aid in digestion and to keep the flora in the digestive tract balanced. Choosing organic foods will decrease your toxin burden while your body is healing. The liver is responsible for producing many of the products necessary for healing. By eating foods lower in toxin burden and foods that support the liver, you will aid your body in recovery.

RECIPES FOR SENSITIVE DIGESTION

Beiler's Broth

Ingredients:
- 1 pound green beans
- 2 pounds zucchini
- 1 bunch regular parsley
- Filtered water, enough to cover all vegetables

Directions:

Bring vegetables to a low boil and continue to boil until very soft. Strain the vegetables into a glass container and keep refrigerated.

> *This broth is highly alkaline and healing. It is often used during acute illnesses and is great to use after a procedure or surgery. During acute distress or post surgery, drink only this broth and water as much as you can through the day for 1–3 days, depending on your situation. When you begin feeling better and think your gastrointestinal tract is ready for solid food, introduce the soft vegetables. Stay gentle on your digestion by eating the soft vegetables at each meal until they are gone. Then you may begin to introduce other foods.*
>
> *As digestion improves but remains sensitive this recipe can be varied in many ways. Onions, garlic, ginger, and seasonings can be added as desired and small amounts of sea salt can also be added. Boiling the vegetables and pureeing them with the water is another way to begin increasing fiber in the diet and testing the gastrointestinal tract for readiness for fiber.*

Simple Smoothie

Ingredients:

½ cup frozen blueberries

½ banana

Filtered water

Directions:

Blend all ingredients in the blender until smooth. This is the simplest form of smoothie. As digestion improves, more fruit can be added, avocado can be included for calories and fat if needed, or protein powders and nutritional powders can be added. As digestion improves, small amounts of fresh spinach can be added for nutrient content.

Pear and Avocado Smoothie

Ingredients:

1 pear

½ avocado

Filtered water

Directions:

Blend all ingredients in the blender until smooth. This smoothie is still very tolerable for most sensitive digestion. As digestion improves, some juice or honey can be added to this smoothie to increase its sweetness.

Banana Avocado Pudding

Ingredients:
   2 bananas
   1 avocado

Directions:
Mix well in blender only until blended and fluffy. Do not over-blend.
Serve chilled and eat immediately.

Savory Squash

Ingredients:
   1 buttercup squash
   2 tablespoons olive oil
   ¼ cup hemp or almond milk
   2 tablespoons honey
   sea salt to taste

Directions:
Cut squash in half and scoop out seeds. Preheat oven to 400° F. Bake
squash in baking pan, sliced side down in 2–3 inches of water for
about an hour or until soft. Remove from the oven, allow to cool
to handling temperature. Scoop meat out into saucepan and add
remaining ingredients. Warm to serving temperature.

Electrolyte Drink

Ingredients:

     2 cups filtered water

     ¼ teaspoon sea salt

     ¼ teaspoon baking soda

     ¼ teaspoon juice of a lemon

     ¼ teaspoon pure maple syrup

Directions:

Mix all ingredients together and drink chilled or room temperature.

> *This is a great alternative to many electrolyte preparations that have significant amounts of sugars and food dyes, which are most likely very acidic. It is helpful in preventing dehydration during times of prolonged diarrhea.*

RECIPES FOR SUFFICIENT DIGESTERS

BREAKFAST
Best Tasting Power Protein Bars

These bars make excellent alternatives for breakfast and snacks on the go. Be careful—these are so good, they're addictive! Also, this recipe tends to vary depending on the liquid content of the almond butter and the quality and texture of the protein powder. You may need to alter the amount of liquid, depending on how the mixture stays together during the hand mixing process.

Ingredients:
 1½ cups rice crisp cereal
 ¼ cup sunflower seeds, half ground
 ¼ cup pumpkin seeds, half ground
 2 tablespoons sesame seeds
 2 tablespoons hemp seeds
 8 scoops or servings protein powder (whey, soy, rice or other
     protein powder alternative)
 ½ teaspoon sea salt
 1½ cups almond butter
 1½ cups brown rice syrup
 1 teaspoon vanilla extract

Directions:
Prepare a greased 9 × 9 or 9 × 13 baking pan or simply line the pan with 2 layers of wax paper. In a separate bowl, mix all dry ingredients together. Warm almond butter and brown rice syrup in a saucepan

over medium heat until soft and fluid. Pour over dry ingredients and begin working mixture with your hands into a large clump. Thoroughly mix the mixture to evenly coat entire dry mix. Press tightly into greased pan or wax paper lined pan and chill in refrigerator until hard. Once hard, cut into squares and store in airtight container. These can very easily be stored in the freezer and taken out a few hours before enjoying.

Gluten-Free Banana Granola Pancakes

Ingredients:

    1½ cups gluten-free pancake or baking mix

    2 bananas, ripe

    1 teaspoon vanilla extract

    ¾ cup hemp milk

    ½ teaspoon baking soda

    ½ teaspoon cinnamon

    1 cup granola

Directions:

Heat lightly oiled skillet to medium heat. Add bananas, milk, and vanilla to blender and blend until smooth. Add baking soda, cinnamon, and half of the baking mix and blend until smooth. Add the second half of the baking mix and blend until smooth. Remove blender, add granola to the mixture and mix in with mixing spoon. Do not blend. Pour batter into 3-inch diameter circles in the pan. When pancakes start to bubble, flip them carefully and cook on the other side until lightly browned on both sides.

Blueberry Syrup

This recipe was given to Dr. Black by Cathe Frederick of Grande Rond, Oregon.

Ingredients:

2 cups organic blueberries

Stevia

Directions:

Take two cups of blended blueberries and strain to remove seeds. Cook on low heat and stir frequently to form a light syrup. Cool slightly and sweeten with pure Stevia to taste. Serve over pancakes or light desserts.

Easy Pancakes with Ground Pumpkin and Sunflower Seeds

Ingredients:

3 tablespoons ground pumpkin seeds

3 tablespoons ground sunflower seeds

3 organic eggs

¼ cup non-gluten flour

¼ cup hemp milk, or other alternative milk

¼ cup uncooked millet (optional)

¼ cup blueberries (optional)

2 teaspoons baking soda

Directions:

Heat lightly oiled skillet to medium heat. Combine all ingredients except blueberries and millet into a medium-sized bowl and mix well until clumps have dissolved. Add blueberries and/or millet if you are going to use these ingredients. Pour batter into 3-inch diameter circles in the pan. When pancakes start to bubble, flip them carefully and cook on the other side until lightly browned on both sides.

SOUPS

Dr. Lang's Healing Soup

Contributed by Renee Lang, N.D.

Ingredients (and benefits to a balanced gut in italics)

   2 tablespoons miso paste (*enzymes, nutrients*)

   1 quart water, filtered (*cleaner and fewer toxins*)

   2 cups organic broccoli, chopped (*nutrient content, fiber, liver support*)

   2 cups organic carrots, chopped (*nutrient content, fiber, liver support*)

   1 tablespoons organic ginger, minced (*anti-inflammatory, digestive aid, liver support*)

   4–6 cloves organic garlic, minced (*anti-oxidant, anti-microbial, liver support*)

   ⅛–¼ cup tamari, to taste (*enzymes, taste*)

   1–2 tablespoons Sesame oil (*taste, a little fat to balance the meal*)

   1 cup quinoa (*excellent source of protein*)

Optional:

   onions minced (*anti-oxidant, vitamin C*)

   turmeric, minced (*anti-inflammatory, anti oxidant*)

   cilantro, minced (*excellent detoxifier, chelator of metals*)

Directions:

Heat water and add miso paste. Do not allow water to boil, but simmer. Allow paste to dissolve. When dissolved, add broccoli, carrots, ginger, garlic, tamari, sesame oil, and quinoa. Cook until vegetables are tender. 30–60 minutes.

Then for easy digestion, and optimal absorption, blend the soup. This will break down the broccoli and carrots even further for ease of digestion.

Taste and add tamari or sesame oil as desired for flavor.

Curry Turmeric Leek Soup

Ingredients:
- 2 leeks, sliced
- 3 tablespoons olive oil
- 1 quart chicken broth
- 5 cloves elephant garlic, sliced into large slices
- ½ head Napa cabbage
- 1 bok choy, chopped
- 1 can diced tomatoes
- 3 teaspoons curry powder or more to taste
- 1 teaspoon turmeric powder
- 1 teaspoon fish sauce
- ½ teaspoon organic lemon juice
- Sea salt to taste

Directions:

Add olive oil to large saucepan or soup pot on medium low heat. Add leeks and elephant garlic and sauté until medium soft. Increase heat to medium and add cabbage and bok choy and sauté for 3–5 minutes. Then add all other ingredients, cover, and simmer on medium to low heat until flavors mingle and vegetables are cooked but still maintain their crunch.

Lentil Apricot Soup

This soup was introduced to Dr. Black by her good friend, Desiree LeFave, a licensed midwife whom she works with often.

Ingredients:

    3 tablespoons olive oil

    1 onion, chopped

    2 cloves garlic, minced

    ⅓ cup dried apricots, minced

    1½ cups red lentils

    5 cups vegetable broth or chicken broth

    3 plum tomatoes, peeled, seeded and chopped

    ½ teaspoon ground cumin

    ½ teaspoon dried thyme

    2 tablespoon fresh lemon juice

    Salt to taste

    Ground black pepper to taste

Directions:

Sauté onion, garlic, and apricots in olive oil. Add lentils and stock. Bring to a boil, then add spices and reduce heat and simmer for 30 minutes, covered and stirring occasionally. Add tomatoes and simmer 10 minutes more. Add lemon juice and puree half of the soup in the blender. Add pureed half back into the soup and serve warm.

SALADS AND RAW

Tabouli

This makes a very pretty dish and always a great dish to bring to a potluck or celebration meal. If you cannot tolerate tomatoes, try replacing them with chopped cucumbers and Kalamata olives.

Ingredients:

1 cup quinoa, cooked and cooled
2 bunches of parsley, regular or flat leaf, minced
1 pint of cherry tomatoes, cut in fours
2–3 cloves garlic, chopped fine
½ cup organic lemon juice
⅓ cup organic cold pressed olive oil
sea salt to taste

Directions:
Start by cooking the quinoa. Add 1 cup of quinoa and 2 cups filtered water to a pan and cover. Bring to boil, reduce heat to medium low and allow to boil/simmer until all the water has been absorbed. Stir occasionally to keep the quinoa from burning on the bottom of the pan. When all the water has been absorbed, remove from heat and allow to cool.

Add cooked quinoa, parsley, garlic, and tomatoes into a large bowel. Pour lemon juice, olive oil and salt over the mixture. Mix well and chill in refrigerator for at least 30 minutes prior to serving. Chilling for at least 24 hours helps the flavors mingle even better.

Kale and Carrot Salad

Ingredients:
>1 bunch kale, chopped
>5 large carrots, sliced
>2 tablespoons sesame seeds
>2 tablespoons hemp seeds
>Sea salt to taste

Dressing:
>1 tablespoon sesame oil
>1 tablespoon olive oil
>⅓ cup brown rice vinegar
>1 teaspoon pure maple syrup

Directions:
Steam carrots and kale until soft but still crunchy and cool. Mix with seeds, coat with dressing mixture, and store in the refrigerator. Flavors will mix if left overnight. Serve chilled.

Easy Salmon Salad

Ingredients:
>2 cans wild boneless, skinless salmon
>½ cup mayonnaise, organic
>½ cup minced carrots
>½ cup minced apples
>¼ cup sweet relish, organic and sweetened naturally

Directions:
Mix all ingredients in a large bowl. Serve chilled with crackers, on a salad, or alone.

Green Drink

> *This is an everyday drink for some of Dr. Black's patients. If you want to use this drink therapeutically, it will cleanse your colon and your blood.*

Ingredients:
  1 bunch parsley
  2–3 cups filtered water
  Lemon juice concentrate to taste
  Molasses to taste

Directions:
Blend on high in the blender until consistency is smooth. It will be frothy, but will reduce as it sits. Drink chilled.

Make this drink and drink ⅓ daily for 3 days in a row and on the fourth day, make a new drink. That way, you only need to make the drink about 2 times per week. For sensitive digestion and if raw foods bother you, begin by drinking only small amounts to gauge your tolerance to the large amount of raw fiber.

ENTREES

Cashew Sauce over Rice, Beans, and Veggies

Ingredients:

- 1 cup brown rice, cooked
- 1 can black beans or ⅔ cup of dry beans cooked with water until soft
- 2 broccoli florets, chopped
- ½ cabbage, chopped
- 3 large carrots, chopped
- 1 bunch kale, chopped

For the Sauce:

- ¼ cup raw cashews, ground to powder
- 1½ tablespoons fresh lemon juice
- 1½ tablespoons nutritional yeast flakes (available at natural food stores)
- 2 teaspoons sweet white miso or ¼ teaspoon salt or tamari to taste
- ½ teaspoon onion or garlic powder
- ¼ cup water (this can be varied depending on how thick you want your sauce to be)
- grated Parmesan cheese to taste (optional, if tolerated)

Directions:

Steam or cook the rice. If using a pan, add rice and 2 cups filtered water to a pan. Bring to boil and allow to boil for 1 minute while stirring, then cover, reduce heat to low and allow to simmer for about 10 minutes or until rice has absorbed the water. Only stir until the heat is reduced to low. While the rice is cooking, prepare the cashew sauce by adding all of the ingredients to a food processor or blender. Blend until smooth. Steam vegetables by chopping them large and adding them to a steaming apparatus. Steam until vegetables are soft but still crunchy. Heat beans in a separate pan.

When preparing to serve this dish, scoop out rice into a bowl, add steamed vegetables and a serving of beans, then top with cashew sauce. This can be added cold or warm.

Hummus

Ingredients:
- 2 cans northern white beans or 1⅓ cup dried beans cooked with water until soft
- ¼ cup liquid from the beans
- ⅓ cup tahini (sesame seed paste found at health food stores or in the Ethnic section of most stores)
- 3 garlic cloves, minced or pressed
- 3 tablespoons filtered water, more or less depending on desired consistency
- ½–1 teaspoon sea salt
- Paprika and olive oil for garnish

Additional ingredients: To make this a nutty/curry hummus, add ½ cup almond butter and 2 teaspoons of curry powder. This is Dr. Black's absolute favorite way to season hummus so it's a must try!

Directions:
Blend all ingredients in a food processor or blender (the blender makes the hummus smoother). Using the white beans in this hummus makes an amazingly smooth and creamy hummus. To serve, pour a small amount of olive oil or white truffle oil over the hummus and garnish with paprika sprinkles. Dip crackers or vegetables in this or spread over toast with avocado.

Coconut Curry Chicken over Brown Rice

This chicken curry requires a little preparation because the chicken is cooked in a crock pot all day prior to the dinner preparation.

Ingredients:

    2 cups rice, cooked

    3–4 chicken breasts

    2 cups water

    1–2 vegetable bouillon cubes, sodium-free

    1 onion, chopped

    3 tablespoons olive oil

    2 broccoli florets, chopped

    ½ head of cabbage, chopped

    3 large carrots, sliced

    1 bag frozen organic peas

    1 can coconut milk

    2 teaspoons curry powder, or more to taste

    1 teaspoon turmeric powder

    1 tablespoon fish sauce

    1 tablespoon pure maple syrup

    Filtered water to taste

    Sea salt to taste

Directions:

Prepare chicken breasts by putting them in the crock pot in the morning with the bullion cubes and 2 cups of water. Cook on low all day. When preparing dinner, begin by cooking the rice. Add rice and 2 cups filtered water to a pan. Bring to boil and allow to boil for 1 minute while stirring, then cover, reduce heat to low and allow to simmer for about 10 minutes or until rice has absorbed the water.

Bring olive oil to medium low heat in a large sautéing pan or wok. Add onion and sauté until soft and translucent. Increase heat to medium and add carrots, cabbage, broccoli, turmeric, and curry powder and sauté until the color in the vegetables is more vibrant. Tease the chicken in the crock pot until it is shredded. Add entire contents of the crock pot and frozen peas to the sautéed vegetables and keep stirring. Reduce heat to low medium and add fish sauce, salt, and coconut milk and continue to cook until flavors mingle but vegetables are still crisp. Serve over cooked brown rice.

Turmeric Lentils with Spinach or Chard

Ingredients:

- 2 cups red lentils
- 4 cups water
- 1 vegetable bullion cube, no salt
- 1 onion
- 2 cloves garlic, minced
- 2 tablespoons olive oil
- 1 tablespoon butter
- 1 tablespoon mustard seeds
- 2 teaspoons turmeric
- ½ teaspoon cumin
- 1 teaspoon coriander
- 1 bunch chard, chopped or 1 large bunch spinach, chopped
- ½ head Napa cabbage (optional)
- 1 lb. seasoned chicken sausage, cooked (optional)

Directions:

In saucepan, add lentils, water, and bullion and bring to boil, covered. Reduce heat to medium low and continue to simmer until all water has been absorbed. This will usually take a little while, so be patient. If all water is absorbed and lentils are not soft, keep adding more water until lentils are soft.

In a separate large saucepan or soup pot, heat olive oil on medium low heat and add mustard seeds for about 1 minute. Make sure to cover with a lid because mustard seeds begin to jump once they are hot. Add onion, garlic, and butter and sauté until soft. Add all spices while stirring and then add chard and cabbage or chicken sausage, if you are including them. Once vegetables are cooked slightly but still crunchy, add lentils and cook a little longer until flavors have mingled. Add sea salt to taste and serve over brown rice or quinoa.

Coconut Brown Rice

Ingredients:
- 2 cups brown rice
- 4 cups filtered water
- 2–3 tablespoons creamed coconut
- ½ teaspoon pure maple syrup

Directions:

Bring rice and water to a boil in a saucepan. Allow to boil for 2 minutes, reduce heat to low, then add coconut and maple syrup, cover, and allow to simmer for 15 minutes. Remove from heat and keep covered for another 5 minutes. Serve warm with your favorite vegetable dish.

Easy Marinade for Chicken, Salmon, or Tofu

Ingredients:
- 2 parts wheat-free Tamari
- 1 part honey
- 1 part dark sesame oil
- Grated ginger
- 1 clove minced garlic

Directions:

Mix all ingredients together. Coat salmon, chicken, or tofu and allow to sit overnight before preparing.

Mushroom Risotto with Cashews and Parmesan

This recipe takes some time to prepare but is definitely worth it! Take the time and you and your guests will be pleasantly impressed.

Ingredients:
    1½ lbs. fresh, wild mushrooms of various kinds (procini, morels, shiitake, Portobello), cleaned, trimmed, and cut into thin strips
    6–7 cups of vegetable or chicken broth
    2 tablespoons olive oil
    1 teaspoon butter
    3 cloves garlic
    1 medium yellow onion, chopped
    1½ cups of Arborio rice
    ⅓ cup Marsala wine
    ⅔ cup dry white wine
    ⅓ cup Parmesean cheese, grated (optional)
    ½ cup ground cashews
    ½ cup chopped flat leaf parsley
    pinch of sea salt to taste

Directions:
Heat the butter and 1 tablespoon of olive oil in a large saucepan over medium heat. Sauté garlic for one minute. Add the mushrooms and sea salt and sauté until the mushrooms release their moisture, get tender, and begin to color around the edges. Heat the remaining tablespoon of olive oil in another saucepan over medium heat and sauté the onion until it is soft and barely golden. At the same time, heat the broth in a soup pan over low heat and keep it warm.

Add the rice to the sautéed onion pan and stir together for a few minutes. Add the Marsala and keep stirring as it reduces, or cooks away. Add the white wine and after it has reduced, stir in the sautéed mushrooms and about one cup of the hot broth. Adjust the temperature to a low medium so that the broth simmers gently with the rice and stir slowly as it reduces. When more than half of the broth has reduced, add another cup of the broth while stirring in the same manner. Continue this process until most of the broth is used and the rice is *al dente*. This will take about 20–25 minutes.

When the rice has reached the right texture, stir in the last cup of broth, Parmesan cheese, and ground cashews and prepare for serving. Right before serving, add the chopped parsley.

Buffalo Steak Marinated in Tequila Lime and Salt

This recipe was inspired by Dr. Black's friend and amazing cook, Rosalinda Camacho in Lafayette, Oregon.

Ingredients:

  2 lb. buffalo steak
  ½ cup tequila
  3 tablespoons lime juice
  1 teaspoon sea salt

Directions:

Add steak and all other ingredients to a small dish or zip lock bag. Rotate often for 24 hours and grill or cook to medium rare.

DESSERT

Coconut Macaroons

Ingredients:

    3 cups unsweetened dried coconut flakes

    1 cup almond meal

    ½ cup raw cacao powder or carob powder

    ½ cup maple syrup

    ¼ cup organic coconut butter

    1 teaspoon organic vanilla extract

    pinch of Himalayan or sea salt

If you don't want to use cacao or carob, you can substitute with another ½ cup of almond meal or coconut.

Directions:

Mix all ingredients together and roll into balls. For a raw dessert, place in dehydrator and dehydrate for 24 hours at a low temperature. To bake, place on greased cookie sheet and bake at 350° for 8–10 minutes.

Almond Cake with Banana, Coconut, and Pineapple Puree

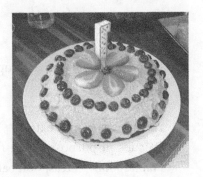

Ingredients:

    2¾ cup almond meal

    2 eggs

    4 tablespoons honey

    ½ teaspoon baking powder

    3 overripe bananas, peeled

    Juice of ½ lemon

    1 teaspoon vanilla extract

    2 cups chopped pineapple

    1 banana

    ½ cup shredded coconut

Directions:

Preheat the oven to 350° F. Generously grease a 9-inch round pie pan. Beat eggs and honey for 10 minutes or until pale and fluffy, then use a fork to mash bananas into this mixture. Add ground almonds and baking powder and stir well. Lastly, stir in the lemon juice and vanilla. Mix until all lumps are dissolved. Pour into baking pan and bake for 45 minutes or until golden brown on the outside and fork inserted in the middle comes out clean. Remove from the oven and leave in pan on a wire rack until completely cooled.

While cooling, add chopped pineapple, coconut, and banana to blender and blend until smooth. Once cooled, insert knife around all edges to loosen the cake. Invert cake quickly onto a flat plate and ease cake out of the pan. Cover with pureed mixture and top with fruit to make a flower decoration.

Vanilla Cake

Ingredients:
   ¾ cup organic butter or 1 cup coconut oil
   1¼ cup honey
   4 large hormone-free eggs
   2 teaspoons vanilla extract
   3½ cups all-purpose gluten-free baking flour
   1 tablespoon + 1 teaspoon baking powder
   1 teaspoon baking soda
   1 teaspoon xanthan gum
   1 teaspoon salt
   1½ cup almond milk

Directions:
Preheat oven to 350° F. Lightly oil 2 8–9 inch round cake pans and dust with gluten-free flour. Melt butter or coconut oil and beat with honey until it becomes fluffy. Lower the speed and add the eggs one at a time while beating. Add vanilla.

In a separate bowl, sift together all dry ingredients. Add half the dry mixture to the wet mixture and beat on low speed until combined. Then add the remaining half of the dry ingredients and beat on low speed until smooth.

Divide batter equally between the two prepared pans. Bake in preheated oven for 35–40 minutes or until a fork can be inserted and comes out clean. Cool the cake for 20 minutes in the pans. Insert a knife around the entire edge loosening the cake from the sides of the pan. Then turn cake over onto wire racks, being very careful when easing the cake out of the pan. Cool completely before frosting.

The two cake layers can be layered on top of each other with or without frosting or filling between the layers.

Honey Vanilla Frosting

Ingredients:
    3 egg whites
    ⅔ cup of honey
    ½ teaspoon xanthan gum
    1 teaspoon vanilla
    pinch of salt

Directions:
Put the unbeaten egg whites, honey, and salt into the top of a double boiler over hot water. Beat with an electric beater on medium to high speed, while you bring the water to a boil. Continue to beat for 7 minutes, or until the mixture forms soft mounds. Remove from the heat, add the vanilla slowly and continue beating until frosting is stiff enough to hold its shape. Wait for the frosting to cool before frosting.

RESOURCES

ONLINE RESOURCES
A Family Healing Center

www.afamilyhealingcenter.com
Drs. Jason and Jessica Black's full-service Naturopathic clinic.

ABC Homeopathy

www.abchomeopathy.com
Great site to learn about homeopathy that also helps you choose remedies on your own if you want learn more.

American Association of Naturopathic Physicians

www.naturopathic.org
National organization of naturopathic physicians; offers some useful information.

Azure Standard

www.azurestandard.com
This is a site where you can order many natural items at a lesser cost than buying in the store. It does have a minimum order, but you can join others who collectively make orders together in your area.

Bastyr University

www.bastyr.edu
Naturopathic medical school located in Seattle, Washington.

The Center for Food Safety: The True Food Network

www.truefoodnow.org
A resource on current eating trends and how to have healthier diet habits.

Centers for Disease Control and Prevention

www.cdc.gov
This is a site that will help you learn more about diseases, prevalence, acute disease outbreaks, vaccinations, and much more.

The Chopra Center

www.chopra.com
A site for learning how to balance the mind, body, and spirit.

Environmental Protection Agency

www.epa.gov
Great site offering current environmental protection advice relating to foods, environmental concerns, and much more. Their mission is to protect human health and the environment.

Environmental Working Group

www.ewg.org wonderful
Wonderful site on environmental toxins and how they are present in our surroundings, and what to do to limit exposure.

Fly Lady

www.flylady.net

A site for helping women to stop procrastinating and for creating better lifestyle habits.

Mayo Clinic

www.mayoclinic.com

A site to learn more about various conditions and the current allopathic approach to those conditions.

National College of Natural Medicine

www.ncnm.edu

Naturopathic medical school located in Portland, Oregon.

National Library of Medicine

www.nlm.nih.gov

Oregon Association of Naturopathic Physicians

www.oanp.org

State organization in Oregon for naturopathic physicians.

RESOURCES SPECIFICALLY FOR DIGESTIVE DISEASES

Australia Crohn's & Colitis Association

www.acca.net.au

Caring Bridge

www.caringbridge.org

Free, personalized websites that connect family and friends during a serious illness. Visit www.caringbridge.org/visit/dedecummings to view Dede's personalized site as an example and read more about her personal journey.

The Crohn's & Colitis Foundation of America

www.ccfa.org

A non-profit, volunteer-driven organization dedicated to finding the cure for Crohn's disease and ulcerative colitis.

Crohn's & Colitis Foundation of Canada

www.ccfc.ca

HealingWell.com

www.healingwell.com

Social network and support community. You'll find information, resources, and support, plus full access to the forums and chat rooms.

Irritable Bowel Syndrome Health Center

www.webmd.com/ibs/default.htm

National Digestive Diseases Information Clearinghouse

digestive.niddk.nih.gov/index.htm

Teens with Crohn's Disease

pages.prodigy.net/mattgreen/

HELPFUL BOOKS AND DVDS

Andersen Wayne Scott, *Dr A's Habits of Health: The Path to Permanent Weight Control and Optimal Health*, Habits of Health Press, 2009.

Dr. Andersen's book has so much useful information about diet and lifestyle support, plus he has an informative website and e-mails newsletters with useful, weekly tips (for example, get up from your desk and stretch, drink water, etc.).

Black, Jessica K., N.D., *The Anti-Inflammation Diet and Recipe Book: Protect Yourself and Your Family from Heart Disease, Arthritis, Diabetes, Allergies, and More*, Hunter House, 2006.

This book offers excellent recipes that are completely hypoallergenic and anti-inflammatory.

D'Adamo, Peter and Catherine Whitney, *Eat Right for Your Type*, Putnam, 1996.

For individuals who do not know what they are intolerant to, or for those extra sensitive individuals who seem to react to odd foods that are not termed, "inflammatory," other diets might be an option. The *Eat Right for Your Type* Diet was developed by Dr. Peter D'Adamo. He scientifically and elegantly describes how certain foods are better tolerated or more aggravating for an individual depending on that person's blood type. He further discusses particular foods that may be a benefit for some blood types, but can be hindering for others. He describes foods, types of exercises, and even condiments and seasonings that are more appropriate for individuals based on their blood type.

Eden, Donna, *Energy Medicine: Balancing Your Body's Energies for Optimal Health, Joy, and Vitality*, Tarcher, 2008.

This is such an excellent book and it can offer many ideas on daily tapping routines to increase the flow of energy in the body and help to make healing possible.

Fallon, Sally, *Nourishing Traditions: The Cookbook that Challenges Politically Correct Nutrition and the Diet Dictocrats*, New Trends Publishing, 1999.
This is a cookbook and an excellent resource if you want to learn how to begin making more home made fermented foods.

Gates, Donna and Linda Schatz, *The Body Ecology Diet: Recovering Your Health and Rebuilding Your Immunity*, Body Ecology 2006.
This book discusses increasing gastrointestinal resistance and overall health by the use of probiotics.

Gershon, Michael D., *Second Brain: The Scientific Basis of Gut Instinct and a Groundbreaking New Understanding: of Nervous Disorders of the Stomach and Intestine*, Harper-Collins, 1998.
A book that explores the enteric nervous system, otherwise known as the brain of the gut, sometimes with humor.

Gottschall, Elaine Gloria, *Breaking the Vicious Cycle: Intestinal Health Through Diet*, Kirkton Press, 1994.
Investigates the link between food and intestinal disorders such as Crohn's disease, ulcerative colitis, diverticulitis, celiac disease, cystic fibrosis, and chronic diarrhea.

Kamm, Laura Alden, *Intuitive Wellness: Using Your Body's Inner Wisdom to Heal*, Atria Books/Beyond Words, 2006.
Laura Alden Kamm endured her own personal health journey and came out on the "other side" in her remarkable memoir.

Kinderlehrer, Jane, *Confessions of a Sneaky Organic Cook or, How to Make Your Family Healthy When They're Not Looking!*, New American Library, 1972.
This is an older book but has so many good ideas in it. Usually you can find one used online for a very inexpensive price.

Lair, Cythia, *Feeding the Whole Family: Cooking with Whole Foods*, Sasquatch Books, 2008.
This is a fun book that gives many ideas on quick meals for the family.

Remen, Rachel Naomi, M.D., *Kitchen Table Wisdom: Stories that Heal*, Riverhead Trade Books, 1997.
Remen is one of a growing number of physicians exploring the spiritual dimension of the healing arts.

Santorelli, Saki, *Heal Thy Self: Lessons on Mindfulness in Medicine*, Three Rivers Press, 2000.
Santorelli, director of the Stress Reduction Clinic at the University of Massachusetts Medical Center, does a wonderful job with this book and it is one of Dede's favorites in aiding her recovery. Santorelli guides the reader through the process of learning to listen to our bodies, and bring mindfulness into our lives. Most of the patients in the Stress Reduction Clinic have never meditated, or been involved in groups or alternative therapies, so his work, and that of the clinic's founder, Jon Kabat-Zinn, is highly regarded and a model of success.

Scala, James, *The New Eating Right for a Bad Gut: The Complete Nutritional Guide to Ileitis, Colitis, Crohn's Disease, and Inflammatory Bowel Disease*, Plume, 2000.
Dr. Scala's book was one of Dede's first purchases at her local used bookstore after diagnosis. His advice and step-by-step dietary guidelines are enhanced by his clear and concise education in eating a healthy diet. A great compliment for a learning library.

Straus, Martha B., *No-Talk Therapy for Children and Adolescents*, by W. W. Norton, 1999.
Straus opens for readers a huge grab bag of gimmicks, gadgets, and games from which to draw resources appropriate to every no-

talk occasion. This book will be useful for parents or caregivers of younger IBD patients who struggle with a lack of language with which to express their emotions.

Weil, Andrew, *8 Weeks to Optimum Health: A Proven Program for taking Full Advantage of Your Body's Natural Healing Power*, Ballantine Books, 2007.
Dr. Weil is one of our "health gurus" and, again, a great book and website resource.

Yee, Rodney. *A.M. and P.M. Yoga.* DVD. Director: Steve Adams. Rating: NR (not rated.)
Yee, Rodney. *Moving Toward Balance: 8 weeks of Yoga with Rodney Yee*, Rodale Books, 2004.
Rodney is Dede's "yoga guru" and arguably one of the most important influences on her improved overall health. Together with his wife, Colleen, he teaches yoga in Long Island at "Yoga Shanti" studio. Rodney continues to be supportive of the mind/body connection in health and well-being, offering encouragement to the authors, as well as to his many students. His website: http://www.yeeyoga.com.

REFERENCES

CHAPTER 2

1. Weil, A., M.D. "What is Leaky Gut?" Ask Dr. Weil, 12 December 2005. Web. 17 March 2010.

CHAPTER 3

1. Taeko, D. and Fujihashi, K. "Type 1 and 2 T Helper Cell-mediated Colitis." *Current Opinion in Gastroenterology* 22.6 (2006): 651–57. Print.

2. Rowe, William A. "Inflammatory Bowel Disease." *EMedicine*. December 28, 2009. Web. April 28, 2008.

3. MacDermott, R.P. "Alterations of the mucosal immune system in inflammatory bowel disease." *The American Journal of Gastroenterology* 31.6. (1996): 907-16. Print.

4. Brown S.J. and Mayer L. "The immune response in inflammatory bowel disease." *The American Journal of Gastroenterology* 102.9 (2007): 2058–69. Print.

5. MacDermott R.P. "Alterations of the mucosal immune system in inflammatory bowel disease." *The American Journal of Gastroenterology* 31.6 (1996): 907–16. Print.

6. Caradonna, L., Ph.D. et al. "Phagocytosis, killing, lymphocyte-mediated antibacterial activity, serum autoantibodies, and plasma endotoxins in inflammatory bowel disease." *The American Journal of Gastroenterology* 95:6 (2000): 1389–1614. Print.

7. Racound, A. "Field of Dreams: Jacksonville Jaguars' Quarterback David Garrard Tackles Crohn's." *Crohn's and Colitis Foundation of America*, 2009. CCFA. Web. June 5, 2006.

8. Sartor, R. "Microbial influences in inflammatory bowel diseases." *Gastroenterology* 134 (2008): 577–94. Print.

9. Sartor, R. "Balfour Therapeutic correction of bacterial dysbiosis discovered by molecular techniques." Published online before print. October 23, 2008. *Proceedings of the National Academy of Sciences.*

10. Sokol, H. et al. "Faecalibacterium prausnitzii is an anti-inflammatory commensal bacterium identified by gut microbiota analysis of Crohn disease patients." *Proceedings of the National Academy of Sciences,* October 21, 2008. Online early edition.

11. Miehsler W, Reinisch W., Valic E., Osterode W., Tillinger W. Feichtenschlager T. "Is inflammatory bowel disease an independent and disease specific risk factor for thromboembolism?" *Gut* 53 (2004): 542–548. Print.

12. SriRajaskanthan R., Winter M. and Muller A. "Venous thrombosis in inflammatory bowel disease." *European Journal of Gastroenterology and Hepatology* 17 (2005): 697–700. Print.

CHAPTER 4

1. Rufo, Paul A. and Bousvaros, A. "Challenges and Progress in Pediatric Inflammatory Bowel Disease." *Current Opinions in Gastroenterology* 23.4 (2007): 406–412. Print.

2. Kuitunen M., M.D., Ph.D, et al. "Probiotics prevent IgE-associated allergy until age 5 years in cesarean-delivered children but not in the total cohort." *Journal of Allergy and Clinical Immunology,* Volume 123, Issue 2, Pages 335–341.

3. Lewis, T., Amini, F. and Lannon, R. *A General Theory of Love.* New York: Random House, 2000. Print.

4. Danese, A. "Elevated Inflammation Levels in Depressed Adults With a History of Childhood Maltreatment." *Archives of General Psychiatry* 65.4 (2008): 409–416. Print.

5. Individualized Medicine. Gerard G., M.D., Lecture. Portland, OR.

6. "Antibiotic Resistance Questions & Answers." *Centers for Disease Control and Prevention.* National Center for Health Marketing, September 16, 2009. Web. November 2009.

CHAPTER 5

1. Scala, J. *The New Eating Right for a Bad Gut.* New York: Penguin, 2000. Print.

2. Pizzorno J.E. and Murray M.T. *Encyclopedia of Natural Medicine* (revised 2nd ed.). CA: Prima Publishing, 1998. Print.

3. Blakeslee, S. "Complex and Hidden Brain in Gut Makes Stomachaches and Butterflies," *New York Times.* January 23, 1996. Web. July 7, 2007.

4. "Overweight and Obesity: Overweight and Obesity Trends Among Adults." *Centers for Disease Control and Prevention.* National Center for Health Marketing, September 16, 2009. Web. December 2009.

CHAPTER 6

1. Blakeslee, S. "Complex and Hidden Brain in Gut Makes Stomachaches and Butterflies," *New York Times.* January 23, 1996. Web. July 7, 2007.

CHAPTER 7

1. "Overweight and Obesity: Overweight and Obesity Trends Among Adults." *Centers for Disease Control and Prevention.* National Center for Health Marketing, September 16, 2009. Web. December 2009.

2. O'Donnell, C.J. and Elosua, R. "Cardiovascular Risk Factors. Insights From Framingham Heart Study." *Revista Española de Cardiología (English Edition)* 61.3 (2008): 299–310. Print.

3. Gouin, J.P., Hantsoo, L.and Kiecolt-Glaser, J. "Immune Dysregulation and Chronic Stress Among Older Adults: A Review." *Neuroimmunomodulation* 15.4-6 (2008): 251–59. Print.

4. Gareau, M., Silva, M.A. and Perdue, M.H. "Pathophysiological Mechanisms of Stress-Induced Intestinal Damage." *Current Molecular Medicine* 8.4 (2008): 274–81.

5. Ranjit, N. Ph.D. et al. "Psychosocial Factors and Inflammation in the Multi-Ethnic Study of Atherosclerosis." *Archives of Internal Medicine.* 167.2 (2007): 174–181. Print.

CHAPTER 8

1. Kuhbler-Ross, E. *On Death and Dying.* New York: Macmillan, 1969. Print.

2. Bullen, T.F. and Hershman, M.J. "Surgery for inflammatory bowel disease." *Hospital Medicine* 64 (2003): 719–23. Print.

3. "Naturopathy in America." *Coalition for Natural Health*. The History of Traditional Naturopathy, Web. March 16, 2010.

4. Pang, J. et al. "Clinical applications of the Zulinqi acupuncture point." *Acupuncture in Medicine*. 17 (1999): 93–96. Print.

5. Hiroyuki H. and Sugimoto, K. "Curcumin has bright prospects for the treatment of inflammatory bowel disease." *Current Pharmaceutical Design* 15.18 (2009): 2087–94. Print.

6. Cheeke, P.R., Piacente, S. and Oleszek, W. "Anti-inflammatory and anti-arthritic effects of yucca schidigera: A review." *Journal of Inflammation*. March 29, 2006. Web. January 2010.

7. Newman H.A., Kummerow, F.A. and Scott, H.H. "Dietary saponin, a factor which may reduce liver and serum cholesterol levels." *Poultry Science* 37 (1957): 42–46. Print.

8. Griminger P. and Fisher, H. "Dietary saponin and plasma cholesterol in the chicken." *Proceedings of the Society for Experimental Biology and Medicine* 99 (1958): 424–26. Print.

9. Heitzman, M.E., Neto, C.C. Winiarz, E., Vaisberg, A.J. and Hammon, G.B. "Ethnobotany, phytochemistry and pharmacology of Uncaria (Rubiaceae)." *Phytochemistry*, 2005 66(1):5-29.

10. Varilek, G.W. at al. "Green Tea Polyphenol Extract Attenuates Inflammation in Interleukin-2–Deficient Mice, a Model of Autoimmunity." *Journal of Nutrition* 131 (2001): 2034–39. Print.

11. Barclay, L., M.D. "Green Tea Drinking Linked to Lower Risk for Distal Gastric Cancer in Women." *Gut.* 58 (2009): 1323–32.

12. Jin, Xi.et al. "Green Tea Consumption and Liver Disease." *Liver International* 28.7 (2008): 990–96. Print.

13. Van Baarlen, P. et al. "Differential NF-κB pathways induction by *Lactobacillus plantarum* in the duodenum of healthy humans correlating with immune tolerance." *Proceedings of the National Academy of Sciences* 106 (2009): 2371–76. Print.

14. Kajander, K. et al. "Clinical Trial: Multispecies Probiotic Supplementation Alleviates the Symptoms of Irritable Bowel Syndrome and Stabilizes Intestinal Microbiota." *Alimentary Pharmacology & Therapeutics* 27.1 (2008): 48–57. Print.

15. Sokol, H. et al. "*Faecalibacterium prausnitzii* is an anti-inflammatory commensal bacterium identified by gut microbiota analysis of Crohn disease patients." *Proceedings of the National Academy of Science* 105: (2008): 16731–36. Print.

16. Schwartz, A.G. and Pashko, L.L. "Dehydroepiandrosterone, glucose-6-phosphate dehydrogenase, and longevity." *Ageing Research Reviews* 3 (2004): 171–87. Print.

17. Bonau, R.A. et al. "High-branched chain amino acid solutions: relationship of composition to efficacy." *Journal of Parenteral and Enteral Nutrition* 8.6 (1984): 622–27. Print.

18. "Study Underway to Find an Alternative Cure for Crohn's Disease and Ulcerative Colitis" *Rush University Medical Center.* News Releases, June 16, 2008. Web. February 2010.

CHAPTER 9

1. Mokdad, A. H. Ph.D et al. "Actual Causes of Death in the United States, 2000." *Journal of the American Medical Association* 291.10 (2004): 1238-1245. Print.

2. AICR and the World Cancer Research Fund. "*Food, Nutrition, Physical Activity and the Prevention of Cancer: a Global Perspective.*" *AICR.* November 2007. Web. December 2009.

3. Bays, H.E. et al. "Prescription Omega-3 Fatty Acids and Their Lipid Effects: Pathophysiology of Hypertriglyceridemia." *Expert Review Cardiovascular Therapeutics* 6.3 (2008): 391–409.

4. O'Keefe, J.H., M.D. et al. "Dietary Strategies for Improving Post-Prandial Glucose, Lipids, Inflammation, and Cardiovascular Health." *Journal of the American College of Cardiology* 51.3 (2008): 249–55.

5. "Mercury Content Labeling Proposed." *Mercury Policy Project.* The Tides Center. Web. March 2010.

CHAPTER 10

1. Eden, D. and Feinstein, D. *Energy Medicine.* New York: Tarcher. 1999. Print.

2. Matsuzaki T. et al. "Mirthful laughter differentially affects serum pro- and anti-inflammatory cytokine levels depending on the level of disease activity in patients with rheumatoid arthritis." *Rheumatology* 45 (2006): 182–86. Print.

3. Chaya M.S. Kataria, M. and Nagendra, R. "The effects of hearty extended unconditional (HEU) laughter using laughter yoga techniques on physiological, psychological, and immunological parameters in the workplace: a randomized control trial." *American Society of Hypertension 2008 Annual Meeting.* May 14, 2008.

4. "Laughter Lowers Blood Pressure." *Laughter Yoga International.* Dr. Kataria. Web. January 2010.

CHAPTER 12

1. Spiegal, J. E. "In a Downturn, a Growth Opportunity." *The New York Times.* February 13, 2009: Page L13. Print..

APPENDIX

1. Shale, M. and Ghosh, S. "Beyond TNF, Th1 and Th2 in inflammatory bowel disease." *Gut* 57 (2008): 1349–51. Print.

2. Berger, A. "Science Commentary: Th1 and Th2 responses: what are they?" *British Medical Journal* 321(2000): 424. Print.

3. Harrington L.E., Hatton R.D., Mangan P.R., Turner H., Murphy T.L., Murphy K.M., Weaver C.T. "Interleukin 17-producing CD4+ effector T cells develop via a lineage distinct from the T helper type 1 and 2 lineages." *Nature Immunology.* 6.11 (2005): 1123–32. Print.

4. "T Helper Cell." *Wikipedia.* Wikimedia Foundation Inc. July 8, 2009. Web. January 2010.

5. Tangye, S. G. et al. "Follicular CD4+ T helper cells induce human B cells to undergo Ig isotype switching and differentiation to Ig-secreting cells through the production of IL-21." *The Journal of Immunology* 95.1 (2007): 178. Print.

6. Shale, M. and Ghosh, S. "Beyond TNF, Th1 and Th2 in inflammatory bowel disease." *Gut* 57 (2008): 1349–51. Print.

7. Conti, H.R. "Th17 cells and IL-17 receptor signaling are essential for mucosal host defense against oral candidiasis." *The Journal of Experimental Medicine* 206.2 (2009): 299–311. Print.

GLOSSARY

Acidophilus: Specific type of probiotic that is present in high quantities in adults.

Allopathic medicine: Typically practiced by medical doctors. It is the use of substances intended to reduce or eliminate symptoms.

Antigen: Any foreign substance that enters the body and stimulates an immune response. Antigens can be micro-organisms or foreign bodies.

Apoptosis: Refers to programmed cell death. If a cell is functioning irregularly or has come to the end of its life, the cell itself will trigger cell death.

Biotherapeutic drainage: The use of remedies to cleanse organs and promote optimal organ function in an effort to cure or reverse the disease process.

C-reactive protein: A marker of inflammation in the body that can be tested easily through a simple blood test.

Cytokine: A small protein released by some cells that plays a part in cell-to-cell communication. Some cytokines stimulate inflammation and others suppress inflammation. The balance of cytokines in the body functions to regulate cell-to-cell communication.

Erythrocyte sedimentation rate (SED rate): A measure of how much acute inflammation is occurring in the body. Can be tested by a simple blood test.

Fistula: An abnormal connection or passageway between two epithelium-lined organs or vessels that normally do not connect. It is generally a disease condition, but a fistula may be surgically created for therapeutic reasons.

Histamine: A chemical released from mast cells that is responsible for local inflammatory responses and allergic reactions, but also plays a part in regular physiological functioning in the gut, in addition to acting as a neurotransmitter.

Hormone: A chemical secreted in the body designed to work on specific tissues causing a regulated and expected result.

Ileum: The final section of the small intestine.

Inflammation: A normal process stimulated by the body to help heal a specific injured area or to help defend against infection.

Interleukins: Proteins secreted mostly by white blood cells that act on white blood cells to regulate inflammation and immune responses.

Large intestine: Consists of the cecum and colon.

Leukocyte: A generic term for any white blood cell.

Lymphocyte: A specific type of white blood cell that helps to regulate and initiate immune and inflammatory responses.

Mast cell: An immune cell responsible for allergic reactions. Many of its actions are unknown though it does play a part in initiating inflammation.

Naturopathic medicine: Complex art and science of using treatments to remove the cause of disease and stimulate healing within an organism.

Neurotransmitter: A chemical that regulates, modulates, and amplifies messages between cells and neurons for communication to the nervous system.

Natural Killer (NK) cells: A type of cytotoxic lymphocyte that acts on other cells by releasing cytotoxic chemicals to kill the offending cell by inducing apoptosis.

Oxygen Radical Absorbance Capacity (ORAC): ORAC content refers to how strong of an antioxidant the supplement is.

Pathogen: An organism that causes disease such as bacteria, virus, or other micro-organism.

Probiotic: A symbiotic organism (mostly bacteria and yeast) that exists in a positive relationship with its host. Probiotics line all mucus membranes in the body and help the body to defend against foreign pathogens.

TNF-alpha: A cytokine that stimulates inflammation and also carries out functions such as growth stimulation and growth inhibition, and has some self-regulating properties. It may have functions that are still poorly understood.

UNDA numbers: Combination medicines made of plant and mineral preparations that have affinity for specific organ systems. The name UNDA was derived from undulating water waves that carry medicine.

APPENDIX A

A DETAILED DISCUSSION ON TNF (SEE CHAPTER 3)

Tumor necrosis factor alpha (TNF-α) is a cytokine involved in systemic and acute phase inflammation. When a mast cell is stimulated, it releases TNF-α, histamine, and other cytokines. Every immune cell has the potential to secrete TNF-α, which plays a role in directing and regulating inflammation, inducing apoptosis (programmed cell death in unhealthy "self" cells), and inhibiting tumor formation and viral replication.

TNF-α becomes important to discuss when studying immunological treatment of IBD because drugs called TNF-α inhibitors improve IBD symptoms. In fact, TNF-α inhibitor use has become widespread now for the treatment of both Crohn's and colitis.[1] There are a number of other chemicals important in the inflammatory cascade such as IL-1, leukotrienes, and prostaglandins, which all promote inflammation. Eating a fatty acid called arachidonic acid, which is found in animal fats, produces leukotrienes and prostaglandins, thus stimulating inflammation. This is most probably the reason that eating a high animal fat diet is associated with many significant poor health outcomes. In order for the body to convert arachidonic acid to these inflammatory cytokines, different enzymes are needed to drive one of the two pathways. The cyclo-oxygenase pathway produces prostaglandins (PGs) and the 5-lipoxygenase pathway produces leukotrienes.

Studying fatty acid synthesis and these two pathways becomes very important in the discussion of inflammation and the use of non-steroidal anti-inflammatory medications (NSAIDs) and fever reducing medications. NSAIDs affect the cyclo-oxygenase enzyme pathway, thereby inhibiting the formation of prostaglandins, which would normally cause pain, fever, and inflammation. Because arachidonic acid is found in high concentrations in meat products, many individuals with significant inflammatory diseases fair well by eating vegetarian.

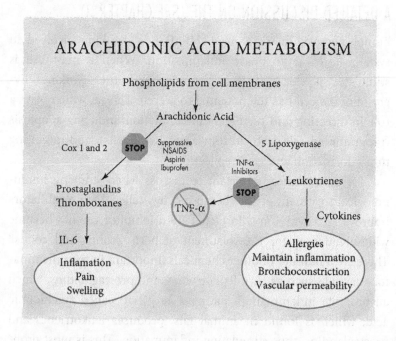

ARACHIDONIC ACID METABOLISM

Phospholipids from cell membranes

Arachidonic Acid

Cox 1 and 2   STOP   Suppressive NSAIDS Aspirin Ibuprofen

5 Lipoxygenase

TNF-α Inhibitors

STOP   Leukotrienes

Prostaglandins Thromboxanes

TNF-α

Cytokines

IL-6

Inflamation Pain Swelling

Allergies Maintain inflammation Bronchoconstriction Vascular permeability

T-LYMPHOCYTES AND THEIR ROLE IN IMMUNE RESPONSE AND INFLAMMATION

The process of inflammation is highly regulated and directed by specific immune cells within the body. As explained earlier, cytokines help to control inflammation through both pro-inflammatory cytokines and anti-inflammatory cytokines. Specific sets of T-lymphocytes drive and direct the immune response based on the type of cytokines they secrete. Two of the main types of lymphocytes are named CD8+ and CD4+ cells. *CD8+ cells* are referred to as cytotoxic cells. About 90 percent of *CD4+ cells* are referred to as T Helper cells and within the small percentage of remaining CD4+ cells, we find regulatory cells such as Treg which act to control or suppress inflammation and mediate immunosuppression. *T Helper cells* can be broken down further into four main categories: Th1, Th2, Th17, and Tfh.[2, 3] All four of these lymphocyte subsets are derived from a naïve T helper cell, TH0, and when in the presence of particular cytokines, they are directed to differentiate into one of the T Helper types and their function becomes highly specific and specialized.

The majority of naïve T Helper cells either become Th1 or Th2 cytokines. *Th1 lymphocytes* are responsible for attack against intracellular pathogens and their response is referred to as cell mediated immunity. *Th2 lymphocytes* are responsible for attack against extracellular pathogens, namely parasites and bacteria and their response is termed humoral, or antibody related, immunity.[4] The balance of these regulatory systems is of extreme importance in protection, injury, and healing. *Th17 lymphocytes* develop on a pathway that is uniquely different than either Th1 and TH2 pathways. Th17 lymphocytes secrete IL-17 and are relatively poorly understood, but rising evidence reveals their connection with mucosal immune system

protection and balance and connection specifically with inflammatory bowel disease.

Tfh cells are the fourth kind of T helper cell and are found in nests
of lymphatic tissue and function to help the B-cells develop into
antibody secreting plasma cells. Tfh cells are needed to direct and
regulate humoral immunity and the Th2 system. Tfh cells secrete a
cytokine named IL-21 and, according to research, may contribute to
the development of immunodeficiencies or autoimmune diseases.[5]

Th1 cytokines are responsible for promoting the inflammatory
response needed for offending against intracellular viruses and
preventing the growth or development of cancer cells, but are also
responsible for autoimmunity and inflammatory related diseases
such as multiple sclerosis, rheumatoid arthritis, ankylosing spondy-
litis, and Sjorgren's. Tissue damage and destruction can occur from
excessive pro-inflammatory cytokine stimulation. The Th2 system
is needed to counteract and provide a balance to the inflammatory
cascade.

This balance can be seen as a scale with the TH1 on one side
of the scale and a TH2 on the other side of the scale. When one
side rises, the other side must lower. This fluctuating dominance
should only change minutely depending on the immune compromise present in order to have the most efficient method of attack to
the offending problem. Although the equilibrium is always dynamic
between these two systems, ideally, the varying difference between
both Th1 and Th2 should never exceed a point in which illness
is caused by the imbalance. Research can't deny that diseases are
not cut and dry, which exaggerates the need for balance between
all Th cell types. Previous analysis of specific immunopathology of
cytokines involved in IBD has most likely supported the concept of
Crohn's as a Th1-dominant disease due to its expression of IL-12 and
IFN-gamma and ulcerative colitis as an atypical presentation of Th2
disease characterized by the production of cytokines such as IL13.

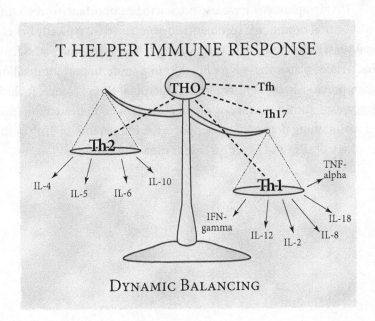

A more recent discovery suggests that the Th17 lymphocyte is a promising target for the cause of IBD and other inflammatory disorders and may be a likelier culprit than the Th1 cell, which was previously believed to be a cause of IBD. Th17 cells are located on the skin and in the gastrointestinal lining and play a role in offending against pathogens. Th17 cells cause attacks on offending organisms by secreting defensins and recruiting other immune scavenging cells such as neutrophils to the site of attack. In essence, the Th17 cells ward off the infection by causing inflammation in the area through the secretion of cytokines, IL-17 and IL-22. This is important because these cells cause inflammation and, if not balanced or regulated, will most likely stimulate inflammatory bowel disease. In fact, to makes things more complicated, recent research in mice has shown a mixed expression of IFN-gamma and IL-17, thus displaying a mixed Th17/Th1 cytokine phenotype, particularly in the gut.[6]

Th17 lymphocytes have also proven to be important in protecting against oral candidiasis (problematic overgrowth of typically beneficial yeast)[7] and because of their strong role in offending pathogenic bacteria, it places these lymphocytes in a more important position than previously thought regarding microbial flora balance, including yeasts, within the mucus membrane. This complicated function of maintaining flora balance supports the importance of Th17 in the etiology of IBD and other gastrointestinal illnesses.

APPENDIX B

TAPPING POINTS FOR FIRST TECHNIQUE OF THE COMMITMENT TO HEAL

(see page 191 for details on the Commitment to Heal)

The first point is at the lateral side of both hands. Using your right hand, lightly karate chop the point on the side of your left hand between the top of your wrist and base of your pinky finger. Keep tapping this point while reciting the statement, "I completely love and accept myself." When finished reciting it one time, lightly tap the same location on your left hand with your right hand, again reciting the statement. You will repeat the statement one time on each tapping location.

The second location is the top of the head. You can find this point by putting the tips of your four fingers from both of your hands on top of your head, meeting your 8 fingers in the middle. Now move the fingers away from each other towards your ears about an inch. Using both hands at the same time, tap lightly on the top of the head, just lateral to midline while reciting the statement one time. When finished, go onto the next point (see the list on page 268) and recite the statement one time, continuing in this fashion until you have gone through all points.

All points are bilateral and will be tapped by the hand on that side of the body simultaneously, except the very first point in which one hand will be tapped first and the other hand will be tapped second.

Tapping locations in tapping order:

    Points 1 and 2: located on the lateral side of both hands between the top of wrist and base of pinky finger

    Point 3: located right at the top of the head, just lateral to midline

    Point 4: located right above the middle of the eyebrow

    Point 5: located right at the temples

    Point 6: located right below the eyes, on the cheek bones

    Point 7: located directly under each nostril, on the upper lip

    Point 8: located right on the chin under the bottom lip, directly in line with point 7

    Point 9: located near acupuncture point Kidney 27. Put your fingers on your clavicle; run them midline until you can feel the larger bumps at the proximal end of your clavicle. Then drop your fingers about an inch lower and slightly outward until they fall into a nice shallow indentation.

    Point 10: located on the side of the body, underneath the armpit. They are horizontally in line with the bra line for women and are horizontally in line with the nipples for men. These points are tapped by bringing both arms up as if to do the chicken dance and allowing the hands to just flop on this area in a comfortable fashion.

    Point 11: located on the lateral side of each wrist where there is a small, soft indentation, Wrist points are done by lightly tapping the wrists together, thereby completing the tapping by bringing the energy back inward creating a closing of the circle.

INSTRUCTIONS FOR SECOND TECHNIQUE
OF THE COMMITMENT TO HEAL

(see page 191 for details on the Commitment to Heal)

1. For this technique, go home and meditate on your core issues. Come up with about five core issues. If you have a hard time coming up with issues, view some of the suggestions below. This may take you a few days to work on, so be patient and trust the thoughts that come to you regarding the emotional issues you need to work on. These core issues can stem from childhood trauma, stress events in the past, etc.

   Core Issue Suggestions:
   I'm not worthy
   I can't have what I want
   I am not good enough
   I don't love, and can't accept, myself
   I am not good enough
   I am a mistake
   I am a failure
   I am abandoned
   I am lost
   I am bad
   I am trapped
   I am a burden
   I am wrong
   I am inadequate

2. Then begin to turn those issues into positive statements and write them down. You might at first think that the positive statement is the exact opposite of what you feel, and that is okay. In fact, if the positive statement is not feeling comfortable for you and you feel it is like lying to yourself, it is a great one to use.

a. For example, "I can't win" or "I can't reach my goals" will become "I can win" or "I can easily accomplish my goals".

b. Make sure that all of the positive statements have positive words. Do not use the words "not", "won't", "no", or any other negative word. Using the sentence, "I am not a burden" is not a good example. The proper sentence to use in this situation would be, "I am worthy" or "I am loved and accepted by others".

c. After all five statements have been given a positive intention, you are ready to go onto the next step.

3. Begin the daily routine by completing one series of the ten tapping points from the first technique described above while reciting the words, "I completely love and accept myself".

4. Now repeat, without tapping, your first core issue positive statement three times with each of the three different beginnings listed below.

a. "I want and I deserve . . . " (i.e . . . *to be loved and accepted by others, to be worthy, to love and accept myself, to honor myself and my gifts*).

b. "I am ready, willing, and able . . . " (i.e . . . *to be loved and accepted by others*).

c. "It is good for me and others, for me . . . " (i.e. *to be loved and accepted by others*).

d. Try to visualize feeling this way. Try to see yourself being loved and accepted by others while you are repeating the sentences.

e. Repeat each 3 beginnings for the next 4 core issues you have listed.

f. If you started with 5 core issues, you should recite 15 sentences.

5. Letting go! After repeating each core issue and its three corresponding positive statements, it is time for forgiveness and release.

   a. Take slow, deep, cleansing breaths and recite a prayer of release and forgiveness.

   You may use any prayer that resonates with you; some people prefer to make up their own prayer or to use a combination of their own words with this example, modified from Henry Lindlahr, M.D.:

   > "I am thankful for being alive and for all the privileges and responsibilities which life confers upon me. I am glad I have another day of glorious opportunity to give and to receive, to gather greater knowledge, and to work for self-completion through better control of all my faculties and powers.
   >
   > I am ready to release any physical and emotional blockages created by my own distorted perceptions.
   >
   > There is that within me which can rise superior to my own weaknesses and to outward circumstances—the power of free will, a spark of the creative force, God, Divine Mind, Holly Spirit, Mother Earth that animates every living being. By the power of the Divine Will within me, I WILL BE WHAT I WILL TO BE. I shall attain complete mastery over my body, mind, and soul; I shall express inward harmony in outward strength, success, and happiness. "

   b. Keep breathing slowly and deeply for a moment after the prayer, visualizing positive health and wellbeing.

6. Make sure to write each core issue down with its 3 new beginnings and repeat all 5 sets of 3 sentences daily. You may want to write each set of 3 positive statements down individually on 5 different note cards or list the fifteen sentences in a row on a piece of paper or in a notebook. It may also be helpful to post these on the mirror in your bathroom to remind you of your worth and to do the technique daily.

7. There is no limit to how many times you can repeat these sentences and prayer daily, but make sure you are visualizing each statement when it is repeated.

INDEX

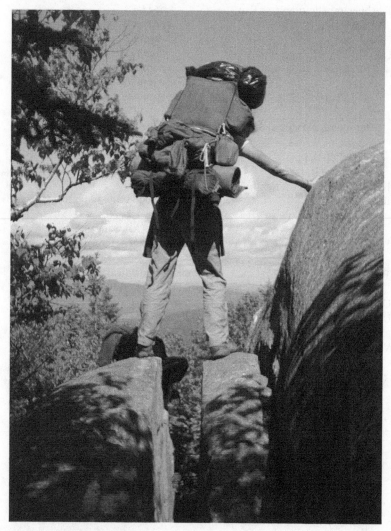

PHOTO BY JOHANNA GARDNER

A FINAL WORD FROM DEDE

CROHN'S AND ulcerative colitis can cause such havoc in one's life, as evident in my story alone; but it is important to note that there is also a redemptive, and comedic, side to this story!

My quest to hike the entire length of Vermont's historic Long Trail began as I lay in my hospital bed at Dartmouth. My roommate had passed away the night before—Mrs. Amidon was in her 90s and she and I bonded during the night after she met with her lawyer that afternoon and got her affairs in order. I was upset the next day and in a great deal of pain. I will never forget what it was like to have a visit from Dr. Bensen, my GI doctor. He sat by my bedside and hung out with me for a while and calmly talked to me about my pain, about moving me to a single room, and about getting well.

My doctor is a physically fit hockey player and coach (in his spare time), who seemed genuinely interested in my outside activities—it turned out we both attended the same undergraduate college (Middlebury) and had lots in common. I shared my love of hiking with him and expressed an interest in hiking Vermont's Long Trail. This was met with an enthusiastic response and thus my goal was stated and is in the process of being attained, section-by-section, in the summers since I have been in remission.

As Dr. Peter D'Adamo said in his wonderful Foreword, to "end your dance on a high note," it is the dance that is the interesting part—the sixty percent of life that *is* the dance, that in fact *leads* to the ending, the high note.

—DEDE CUMMINGS

ACKNOWLEDGMENTS

WE COULD not have done this without tremendous help and support from our families, friends, colleagues, and other newfound heroes in our lives. We wish to acknowledge the following people for their invaluable help in getting this book written, edited, and finally published!

First, and foremost, we would like to thank our publisher, Andrew Flach, for his unflagging support and for believing in our book. Our editorial team was superb: editors June Eding and Anna Krusinski, along with support from Julia Luster, Rachel Schles, and Ryan Tumambing of Hatherleigh Press, helped make this book truly great.

Dede would like to thank Steve, Sam, Emma and Joey Carmichael and her parents, Shirley Ellis Cummings and the late Robert Cummings; along with the following people: Steven Bensen, M.D., Horace F. Henriques, M.D., Peter Banks, M.D., Jeffry Potash, M.D., Renee Lang, N.D., Samantha Eagle, N.D., Jody Noe, N.D., Remeline Damasco, M.D., Laura Metsch, M.D., Greg Gadowski, M.D., John Bookwalter, M.D., Wayne Scott Andersen, M.D., Peter Gibbons, M.D., Gary Clay, M.D., Catherine Dianich Gruver, Lynne Weinstein, Martha Straus, Ph.D., Michael Fleming, Billy Straus and the staff and volunteers of Rescue Inc., Kim Timlege, Ken Steir, Deborah Feiner, Janet Sinclair, Laura Alden Kamm, Rodney Yee, Peter Rizzo, Saki Santorelli, Robin Westen, Elisabeth Gardner, Lisa Mendelsund, Danny Lichtenfeld, Margaret Shipman, Eric Aho, Lee Hill, Julie Ewing, Nan Starr, Marcie, Alex, and Ann Cummings, Jean C. Ellis, Bevin, Martin, Lea and Stacy Carmichael, Lisa

Gruenberg, M.D., Margaret Wimberger, Molly Raymond, Annie Hartman Philbrick, Trina Kassler Waters, my hiking buddies— Amelia Darrow, Johanna Gardener, Anne Latchis, Sharon Snider, Lissa Weinman, Linda Whelihan, Carolyn Kasper, Janice Warren, Maria Chambers, Elizabeth Ungerleider, and Christie Herbert; my musician friends—Bill Conley, John Ungerleider, Tom Grasso; Tom Clynes, Cathy Mizgerd, Lauren and Konstantin von Krusenstiern, Bahman Mahdavi; and other friends, and colleagues who have helped me along the way—John Elder, David Price, Galway Kin- nell, Wyn Cooper, Richard Silverman, William Osono Sirkobei, Dodie Woodbridge, Tanya Tabachnikoff, Shelley Dresser, Kristin Brown, Alan Metcalfe, Margy Klaw, Billy Gordon, John Bell, Judy Whisnant, Pete Gang, Henry Pitney, Geof Fitzgerald, Ellen Starr, Sally and Ricahrd Wiswall, Lisa Van Dusen, Pete Gang, Hester Buell, Len Carr, John Tobin, Megan Hunt, Karen Behringer, Michael Cohen, Ellen Keelan, Cindy Coble, Julie Emond, PT, Rebecca Jones, M.D., Jennifer Pennoyer, M.D. and staff, Suzanne Kingsbury, Mary Alice Hanford, Julie Silver, M.D.; Alison Rosenfeld, Ariella Levine, Bethanne Packard and Chris Mullins at CCFA; Kimberly Allison, M.D., Constance Cummings, Ph.D., Emeran Mayer, M.D., everyone at the Foundation for Psychocultural Research in LA, along with the staff and nurses at Brattleboro Memorial Hospital, Biologic Integra- tive Healthcare, and Dartmouth-Hitchcock Medical Center.

༄

Jessie wants to thank George Bynum, a friend of mine, in advance because I know he will be carrying our book around the country with him showing it to doctors for the next year!

I am thankful to my staff, Judy, Sarah, Diane, and Carolyn for understanding my deadlines and for striving for a smooth function- ing clinic to ease stress and allow more time for me to focus on my book. I am so thankful for all of my patients who make this wonderful knowledge possible and for inspiring me to write this helpful treatment guide.

I am thankful to Dr. Peter D'Adamo for trusting in me and my expertise and for adding such great content to our story.

I am thankful to Alice Black and Ruth Taylor, my husband's mother and grandmother, who have helped take the girls if needed and who moved to Portland so that we could have family closer. I am thankful to my dad, Richard Knabel, for believing in me, supporting me through business decisions, and spreading the word of my expertise with those around him.

I am thankful to my mom, Sandy Stock, for initiating my interest in the complexities of the gastrointestinal tract. She has always believed in me and always has supported me to follow my own path. I am thankful to Cliff Stock, my dad since I was 10, for teaching me about life, helping me through tough struggles that made me grow as a person and to both of them for helping me build confidence from a young age.

I am thankful also to my wonderful friend and nanny, Amity Dehoff, who has helped in every way imaginable around my home and with our family; always working hard to help us maintain a clean, organized, loving, and healthful home. We are all so thankful to have her as a part of our family.

I am so thankful to my husband and my girls for supporting my time commitments to this project. I especially want to thank my eldest, Sadie for the many afternoons we sat side by side, me working and her watching movies, knitting, or reading. I want to thank my youngest, Zienna, for her enduring spunk and energy that she adds to our family. I can't say enough about my husband, Jason, who always inspires and supports me. I look up to him in many ways and admire him as a parent, a physician, a friend, and most of all, my life partner.

ABOUT THE AUTHOR,
JESSICA BLACK, N.D.

DR. JESSICA BLACK graduated from the National College of Naturopathic Medicine where she obtained her medical training. In 2006, Dr. Black published *The Anti-inflammation Diet and Recipe Book,* which is sold internationally and in local bookstores. She now enjoys promoting her book and giving educational lectures in her community. Dr. Black has also published articles in various nutrition magazines.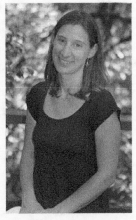

Dr. Black also divides her time between her two Oregon clinic locations offering family health care to Portland, McMinnville, and surrounding counties. She specializes in women's medicine and natural hormone balancing for menopause, as well as childhood wellness including gastrointestinal issues, chronic asthma and acute and chronic illness in children. Because of her thirst for knowledge, she continues to study and research vaccinations, hormones, new treatment ideas, and cutting edge techniques used to improve health. She is currently working on two new books: the first covering childhood development, vaccinations, nutrition, and at-home treatments and a second one covering inflammation, diet and recipes, chronic illness, and disease prevention.

Dr. Black enjoys spending time with her husband, Dr. Jason Black, and their two beautiful and spirited daughters. They love to experiment with fun food and drink creations and celebrate life with friends and family. Dr. Black also enjoys skiing, traveling, biking, and spending time in nature.

ABOUT THE AUTHOR, DEDE CUMMINGS

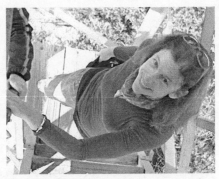

DEDE CUMMINGS, author and Crohn's patient, has been a book designer for the past 25 years. She holds a BA from Middlebury College in Literature. Her hobbies include hiking, yoga, running, reading, gardening and backcountry skiing. Dede has been published by *Family Fun* and *Mademoiselle* magazine and the Crohn's and Colitis Foundation's *Newsletter*. She was a *Discovery/The Nation* poetry semi-finalist, and currently writes in a salon hosted by the author Suzanne Kingsbury.

Dede is a 2010 graduate of the Harvard Medical School's Department of Continuing Education course "Publishing Books, Memoirs and Other Creative Non-Fiction," under the direction of Julie Silver, M.D.

Dede lives in Brattleboro, Vermont, in a house built by her husband, Steve Carmichael. They have three children, Sam, Emma, and Joey. After Dede's most recent hospital stay and surgery for Crohn's disease in 2006, she began hiking the Long Trail (the length of Vermont) in one week sections, beginning to realize a long-term goal that had been put off due to illness.

Visit the the authors' website at
http://www.livingwithcrohnsandcolitisbook.com

A RESOURCE FOR RESEARCH, EDUCATION, AND SUPPORT: THE CROHN'S & COLITIS FOUNDATION OF AMERICA

The Crohn's & Colitis Foundation of America is a non-profit, volunteer-driven organization whose mission is to cure Crohn's disease and ulcerative colitis, and to improve the quality of life of children and adults affected by these diseases. It was founded in 1967 by Irwin M. and Suzanne Rosenthal, William D. and Shelby Modell, and Henry D. Janowitz, M.D. Four decades ago, the Crohn's & Colitis Foundation created the field of Crohn's disease and ulcerative colitis research. Today, the Foundation funds cutting-edge studies at major medical institu¬tions, nurtures investigators at the early stages of their careers, and finances underdeveloped areas of research. In addition, the Foundation provides up-to-date information on Crohn's disease and ulcerative colitis to educate the community while providing critical support to patients and their loved ones.

Call 888.MY.GUT.PAIN or visit the CCFA's website at http://www.ccfa.org for more information on the Foundation's research, education, and support initiatives.

NOTES FROM YOUR DOCTOR/GI CLINIC